Obstructed Labour

Sheryl Nestel

Obstructed Labour:
Race and Gender in the Re-Emergence
of Midwifery

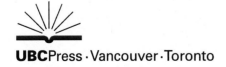
UBCPress · Vancouver · Toronto

16 15 14 13 12 11 10 09 08 07 06   5 4 3 2 1

Printed in Canada on ancient-forest-free paper (100% post-consumer recycled) that is processed chlorine- and acid-free, with vegetable-based inks.

Library and Archives Canada Cataloguing in Publication

Nestel, Sheryl, 1950-
  Obstructed labour : race and gender in the re-emergence of midwifery / Sheryl Nestel.

Includes bibliographical references and index.
ISBN-13: 978-0-7748-1219-1 (bound); 978-0-7748-1220-7 (pbk)
ISBN-10: 0-7748-1219-2 (bound); 0-7748-1220-6 (pbk)

  1. Midwifery – Social aspects – Ontario. 2. Minority women – Ontario. 3. Discrimination in medical care – Ontario. 4. Sex discrimination against women – Ontario. I. Title.

RG950.N47 2006   618.2'0089   C2005-906964-3

Canadä

UBC Press gratefully acknowledges the financial support for our publishing program of the Government of Canada through the Book Publishing Industry Development Program (BPIDP), and of the Canada Council for the Arts, and the British Columbia Arts Council.

This book has been published with the help of a grant from the Canadian Federation for the Humanities and Social Sciences, through the Aid to Scholarly Publications Programme, using funds provided by the Social Sciences and Humanities Research Council of Canada.

Printed and bound in Canada by Friesens
Set in Stone by Artegraphica Design Co. Ltd.
Copyeditor: Anne Holloway
Proofreader: Judy Phillips
Indexer: Christine Jacobs

UBC Press
The University of British Columbia
2029 West Mall
Vancouver, BC V6T 1Z2
604-822-5959 / Fax: 604-822-6083
www.ubcpress.ca

Contents

Acknowledgments / vi

Acronyms / viii

Introduction: A New Profession to the White Population in Canada / 3

1 Technologies of Exclusion / 17

2 Midwifery in Ontario: A Counter-History / 37

3 Midwifery Tourism / 69

4 "Ambassadors of the Profession": The Construction of Respectable Midwifery / 84

5 Narratives of Exclusion and Resistance of Women of Colour / 125

Conclusion: The Construction of Unequal Subjects / 160

Appendix A: Information letter for research participants / 167
Appendix B: Poster to solicit study participants / 168
Appendix C: Chronology of midwifery in Ontario / 168
Appendix D: Interview for immigrant midwives of colour / 169
Appendix E: Interview for white "non-elite" midwives / 169
Appendix F: Interview for white members of midwifery bodies / 170
Appendix G: Interview for women of colour who participated on
                     midwifery bodies / 170

Notes / 171

References / 182

Index / 196

Acknowledgments

I am indebted to many people for their support. My community of friends at the Ontario Institute for Studies in Education of the University of Toronto, many of them activist/scholars of dedication and accomplishment, provided a rich and supportive environment. Thanks especially to Yvonne Bobb-Smith, Jane Ku, Eve Haque, Amina Jamal, Lorena Gajardo, Nuzhat Amin, Janice Hladki, Zoe Newman, and Doreen Fumia. They have always been there to listen, read, critique, and celebrate, all in good measure. Esther Geva and Cheryl Gaster have provided sound advice, encouragement, and Shabbat dinner. Friends outside of academia have offered unerring support, happy distraction, and intelligent feedback. Thanks especially to Rhonda Chorney, Isabella Meltz, Anona Zimerman, and Jaye Rosen. Thanks also to Claire Pizer for helping me live through this. Emily Andrew, my editor at UBC Press, is the epitome of professionalism and has made a potentially unnerving process almost painless.

Lesley Biggs and Patricia Kaufert have offered wonderful feedback and support. Thanks to Ivy Bourgeault for writing the thesis that provided a roadmap to the re-emergence of midwifery, and for many hours of good talk. Christine Sternberg, RM, has been a sounding board, a critical reader, and walking proof that resistance is always possible. Sara Booth, RM, has been a mainstay throughout this project, urging me on through moments of painful uncertainty.

This book began as doctoral thesis, and I had the good fortune to have supervision from a most extraordinary trio. Kari Dehli has maintained a constant interest in my work and urged me to take it in new directions. Ruth Roach Pierson is a scholar to be emulated, a steady ally, and a joyful presence. She has mentored me and nurtured me in innumerable ways, and I treasure our friendship. I was honoured that Inderpal Grewal agreed to serve as my external examiner, and I am grateful for her participation and her comments. My supervisor and dear friend Sherene Razack is a woman of extraordinary generosity, acute intelligence, and keen observation. All of us who work and celebrate life with her derive enormous benefit from her finely honed sense of justice and from her ability to recognize what is really important in life. In the thirteen years I have known and worked with her, she has never let me down.

My dear friends Donna Jeffery, Barbara Heron, and Carol Schick have provided emotional and intellectual sustenance with unstinting dedication; I am privileged to receive the bounty of their friendship. My husband, Sydney Nestel, has remained unflappable throughout these years of trying to balance work, graduate education, and family. He is my best critic and most steadfast support, and I thank him with all my heart. My children Yona, Hadar, and Yehuda have generously cheered me on, and nothing has been more gratifying for me than watching them develop their own commitment to social justice. My mother, Flo Baron, has been supportive throughout the long process of bringing this book to publication.

Material support is crucial and I am grateful to the Social Sciences and Humanities Research Council of Canada for awarding me doctoral and postdoctoral fellowships.

Brenda Hyatali, a woman of extraordinary courage, optimism, and kindness, made the conceptualization and completion of this book possible and I dedicate it to her.

Portions of the introduction and of Chapter 1, Technologies of Exclusion, were previously published in *Health and Canadian Society/Santé et Société Canadienne* 4, 2 (1996-97): 351-41, and appear here in a revised and updated form. In addition, Chapter 3, Midwifery Tourism, first appeared in the *Canadian Journal of Law and Society/la Revue Canadienne Droit et Société* 15, 2 (2000): 187-215. It too appears here in a revised form.

Acronyms

AOM   Association of Ontario Midwives
CAC   Community Advisory Council (to the Prior Learning Assessment Program)
CDC   Curriculum Design Committee on the Development of Midwifery Education in Ontario
CDN   Canadian dollars
CMO   College of Midwives of Ontario
HPLR   Health Professions Legislation Review
IRCM   Interim Regulatory Council on Midwifery (Ontario)
MEP   Midwifery Education Program
MIPP   Midwifery Integration Planning Project
MTFO   Midwifery Task Force of Ontario
OAM   Ontario Association of Midwives
ONMA   Ontario Nurse-Midwives Association
OSCE   Objective Structured Clinical Examination
PLA   Prior Learning Assessment
PLEA   Prior Learning and Experience Assessment
RHPA   Regulated Health Professions Act
RM   Registered Midwife
TCCMO   Transitional Council of the College of Midwives of Ontario
TECMI   Toronto East Cultural Mentorship Initiative
TFAPTO Task Force on Access to Professions and Trades in Ontario
TFIMO   Task Force on the Implementation of Midwifery in Ontario
TOEFL   Test of English as a Foreign Language
VON   Victorian Order of Nurses

Obstructed Labour

Introduction: A New Profession to the White Population in Canada

> How do you get to be the sort of victor who can claim to be the vanquished also?
>
> – Jamaica Kincaid, *Lucy*

In November of 1987, Betty-Anne Putt, practising midwife and active member of the Association of Ontario Midwives, addressed a conference convened in Montreal in support of the shift of Aboriginal health programs to the control of First Nations authorities (Association of Ontario Midwives 1988).[1] Putt, a non-Aboriginal woman, urged the participants to reject the medical practices of "the white man's institutions" and to return to "practices closer to [First Nations] culture and spirit." Identical intentions, she claimed, had shaped the re-emergence of midwifery in Ontario, where women had striven to move childbirth closer "to the way *our* ancestors did it" (emphasis in the original). Women's lobbying and political action, Putt explained, had led to government recommendations designed to protect "normal" birth, and to the creation of a "new profession to the white population in Canada" (AOM 1988, 8).

Putt's remarks are both highly problematic and unwittingly accurate. Problematic is her portrayal of Aboriginal cultures as static and curiously unaltered by centuries of colonization and genocide. Equally troubling is her contention that white women and First Nations people have been victimized in parallel ways by "white man's institutions" – a disturbing erasure of the ways in which white women both benefit from race privilege and have participated in racial dominance. Rey Chow (1993, 13) finds such discursive strategies to be a form of "self-subalternization which draws on notions of lack, subalternity, [and] victimization" to gain authority and power for dominant subjects. Unwittingly accurate, however, is Putt's description of the re-emergence of Ontario midwifery in the last two decades as the creation of "a new profession to the white population in Canada." "In creating a movement," admitted one midwifery activist, "white, educated, able-bodied, middle-class women have tended to attract the same, leaving many voices behind" (Ford 1992, 50).

Among the "voices" that have been left behind are the hundreds, if not thousands, of immigrant women of colour who possess formal midwifery credentials from their countries of origin in the global South. Their meagre representation among registered midwives in the province represents a clear paradox. "Visible minority" people account for approximately 19 percent of Ontario's total population (Statistics Canada 2003). In Toronto, histori-cally the centre of midwifery activism, they account for 44 percent of all residents (Statistics Canada 2004). However, the number of midwives of colour expressing an interest in having their credentials recognized in the province has, since 1986, outstripped their proportion in the population at large, accounting for nearly half of those who, by 1994, had sought infor-mation from the College of Midwives and its predecessors about credentials assessment (Task Force on the Implementation of Midwifery in Ontario 1987, 331; College of Midwives 1994a). Relatively few of these women have suc-ceeded in becoming registered as midwives.

Integration into the midwifery profession, by all available routes, of both immigrant midwives of colour and other racialized women has been, and continues to be, a protracted and problematic process.[2] Prior to the gradua-tion in September 1996 of the first class of the baccalaureate-granting Mid-wifery Education Program, only one out of the seventy-two registered midwives in Ontario was a woman of colour. By December 1996, there were ninety-two registered midwives of whom three (3.3 percent) were women of colour. By May 1998, there were 126 registered midwives, among whom were twelve women of colour and one First Nations woman, bringing the percentage of non-white midwives to 10.3 percent. While it was reported by one College of Midwives of Ontario official that in 1998 46 percent of the PLEA graduates and 13 percent of the midwifery education program were women of colour (Tyson 2001, 13), the percentage of these women who have actually become registered remains at approximately 12 percent (Ford and Van Wagner 2004, 258).[3] This book seeks to capture elements of racial exclusion as they played out during the most formative years of the re-emergence of midwifery, spanning the early 1980s through the end of 1998. Relatively recent changes notwithstanding, such as the streamlining of the process aimed at integrating internationally trained midwives and other professionals, a considerable history of exclusion within the midwifery move-ment in Ontario preceded the current concern with equitable practices in the recognition of international credentials.

The picture that emerges is one of a predominantly white midwifery ap-paratus in a province whose multiracial character is one of its most fre-quently invoked social signifiers (Abate 1998, A6), as well as one in which immigrant midwives of colour are in abundant supply. The processes that (re)produce racially exclusive spaces result from both deliberate choices and from seemingly benign inertia, but neither of these is necessarily linked to an intention to enact racism. Rather, racist exclusion must be understood as unavoidable when race-blind epistemologies guide actions. The assumption that guided Ontario midwifery was that women were oppressed in similar ways and that race, class, and sexuality only complicated a fundamental gender oppression. Such a stance does not require that relations of domination *between* women be taken into account, and thus a path is cleared for racial domination to be re-enacted within a feminist context. The Ontario midwifery movement understood its project as one that benefited all women equally. That women's stakes in the politics of midwifery – whether as providers or consumers of midwifery care – reflected the ways in which they were positioned by race was not taken into consideration. The inevitable result was racist exclusion.

As a project that aimed to address the "universal needs of women" (Glenn 1992, 37), the midwifery movement in Ontario required a universal woman as the protagonist of its "heroic tale," in which autonomous subjects, constrained only by gender inequity, pursue and win their goal through dedication and courage. As is often the case when gender-based paradigms reign, that universal woman "embodies the characteristics of the most privileged women" (Razack 1998a, 340). Engagements with subordinate groups such as First Nations women and immigrant women secured rather than challenged such privilege. From its inception, midwifery's self-definition and the material requirements for participation in the Ontario midwifery movement worked to define immigrant midwives of colour as being on the margins (if not outside) of the movement's perimeter. They posed both a material and symbolic threat to the heroic tale and to its victorious resolution through legalized midwifery. An initial unease with the threat of immigrant midwives of colour entering the movement escalated into a full-blown set of discriminatory structures that facilitated their exclusion from practice after the legislation was passed.

Many births throughout the world are attended by midwives trained in a variety of ways that range from traditional apprenticeship models to models grounded in Western medical and obstetrical knowledge, to models that borrow liberally or judiciously from each of these. In North America, however, physicians have maintained a century-long monopoly over care to pregnant and birthing women. The medical model within which physician care has been offered has historically regarded human parturition as an inherently risky and often pathological process. While childbirth-reform activists have long argued that many standard obstetrical procedures are both inhumane and clinically ineffectual, such practices have been slow to disappear (Enkin, Keirse, and Chalmers 1995; Kaczorowski et al. 1998). One response to the medicalization of childbirth in North America has been the revival over the last thirty years of the practice of community-based midwifery, which provides services to birthing women outside of conventional medical institutions. While the practice of "lay midwifery," with a few exceptions, was largely eradicated in Canada early in the twentieth century, in the 1970s it began to be embraced by some middle-class white women (Fynes 1994).[4] These empirically trained midwives acquired the necessary skills within a framework that promoted informed choice in the birthing process, appropriate use of technology, and the recognition of birth as a psychosocial as well as a physiological event. Central to this form of midwifery has been the belief that women have a fundamental right to choose where they give birth and that the home is the birthing venue most likely to provide the setting for humanized childbirth. Decidedly white and middle class, the midwifery movement in Ontario grew from these roots and incorporated aspects of feminist and traditional women's health movements, counterculture lifestyle practices, and long-standing efforts by white British-trained midwives to have their skills recognized within the health care system.[5] By the mid-1980s, midwifery shifted from a loosely organized social movement to a tightly orchestrated political project that systematically pursued state regulation and funding for the revitalized profession (Van Wagner 2004).

The first Canadian legislation establishing midwifery as a state-regulated and state-funded health profession was passed into law in Ontario on 31 December 1993. Hailed as a "victory for women" (D. Martin 1992, 417), the enactment of midwifery legislation in Ontario has been viewed as a triumph of grassroots feminist organizing and as part of the ongoing struggle for gender equity and female reproductive autonomy. The midwifery model of practice as developed in Ontario has much to recommend it over a medical model of maternity care that has been documented as consistently overly interventionist and frequently misogynistic (Davis-Floyd 1992; Rothman 1982; E. Martin 1992; Oakley 1984; Scully 1994).[6] However, the benefits resulting from the legalization of midwifery have been very unevenly distributed. Like many other feminist projects of the last three decades that have claimed to seek gains for all women, the Ontario midwifery movement has produced economic and sociopolitical rewards primarily for white women.

The role of law in creating racialized subjects has been crucial. The legislation distinguishes between legal and illegal midwives but leaves these classifications relatively unspecified. Their character has instead been transformed through the process by which the Midwifery Act has been implemented. Those empowered by law to develop the disciplinary framework of the profession made decisions early on that served to racialize the "illegal" category.

In the province of Ontario, immigrant midwives of colour who possess considerable professional skills, competencies, and credentials have found themselves largely excluded from access to the newly legalized midwifery profession.[7] While in the period immediately following legalization, racialized minority women represented nearly half of the hundreds of women who had inquired about having their prior midwifery training recognized in the province, as noted above, they currently comprise just 12 percent of registered midwives in the province. The devaluing of non-European experience, credentials, and training; the deployment of inferiorizing discourses surrounding "immigrant women"; a tenacious adherence to forms of feminist politics that privilege the skills and interests of white women; and numerous acts of "everyday racism" (Essed 1991) have converged to create a predominantly white midwifery profession.

Those seeking legal status and state funding for midwifery in Ontario were faced with the task of constructing an authoritative political identity in a sociopolitical context where physicians regarded midwives with more than a modicum of ambivalence.[8] Despite the legalization of the profession in a number of Canadian provinces, midwifery continues to be perceived as an archaic and discredited form of maternity care or as a primitive practice surviving only in "underdeveloped" regions.[9] As one recent study shows, the *Canadian Medical Association Journal* ceased publishing articles that represented midwives as atavistic relics only after midwifery legislation was passed in Ontario (Winkup 1998). Such ambivalence is not limited to doctors. Vilified for much of the last century, the midwife has been portrayed as a degenerate and unmistakably racialized figure in both professional medical journals and popular writing (women's magazines, pregnancy advice literature, etc.), and her "primitive" ministrations were contrasted with the "advances" of medical science. For the midwifery project to achieve broad-based political support, the midwife needed to be reconfigured in the public imagination as respectable, that is, knowledgeable, modern, educated, and Canadian/ white. Women whose identities endangered this reconfiguration often faced expulsion from the midwifery "sisterhood."

In Ontario, a place significantly shaped in the last three decades by postcolonial migrations, these racially exclusionary dynamics reflect not only histories of colonialism, but contemporary relations of domination where the local and the global are so thoroughly intertwined that their status as oppositional categories can no longer be defended (Said 1993; Stoler 1995). Liberation movements are not exempt from enmeshment in such neocolonial processes, and the movement to legalize midwifery in Ontario offers a paradigmatic example of this. Like many feminist projects of the nineteenth and twentieth centuries, it occupies a "historically imperial location" (Burton 1994, 1), deriving material and discursive benefit from an engagement with Third World women.[10] While midwifery policies and every-day practices in the province have discouraged the entry of immigrant women of colour into the newly prestigious profession, travel to the Third World and access to the bodies of birthing women there have played an indispensable role in the legalization of midwifery by helping white mid-wives achieve professional knowledge and status.[11] These travels are ren-dered benign and even benevolent through claims about women's shared identity, an alchemical process in which Third World space and those who occupy it come to constitute a commodity for First World women's con-sumption and social advancement.

This study focuses on a very specific feminist initiative – the movement to revive the practice of midwifery in Ontario, Canada – and pivots on sev-eral key questions:

- How have legacies of colonialism, including an increasingly globalized economy, structured the conditions under which white women in the West transform their relationship to patriarchal forms of social organization?
- How are feminist projects that make claims on the state regulated in ways that reproduce racial dominance through legal and institutional means?
- How are practices of racist exclusion implemented in such projects through the privileging of white cultural competencies?
- How and to what extent do members of dominant groups fail to recog-nize such exclusionary practices as racialized forms of power?

In the course of this research, hundreds of documents and publications linked to the development of midwifery in Ontario between 1981 and 1998 have been examined and analyzed. These documents, which came from both the Ontario midwifery movement and the provincial government, were supplemented with interviews conducted with white members of the Task Force on the Implementation of Midwifery (the first government body established to shape the criteria for entry to the new profession in the prov-ince), with white members of the Interim Regulatory Council on Midwifery (the successor body that formulated regulatory policies prior to legaliza-tion), and with officials of the College of Midwives of Ontario. I have inter-viewed relatively few white women who participated at the policy-making level in either midwifery organizations or government-appointed bodies related to the re-emergence of the profession, mainly because the ideologies and political positions of such women have been widely circulated in the documents reviewed. I have examined these not only to locate the deci-sions that have effected exclusions, but also to uncover the "discursive rep-ertoires" evident in the texts, as well as in the collected narratives, which demonstrate the many ways in which racist exclusion is named, justified, and rationalized as something other than subordination (Wetherell and Potter 1992, 2).

Global and institutional processes link inextricably with numerous microprocesses that differentiate "respectable" midwives from those practitioners deemed unworthy of inclusion in the new profession. My research examined these processes at work among three groups: white midwives who defined themselves as socially, politically, or ideologically estranged from the central group of midwives who orchestrated much of the legalization project; students in the provincial Midwifery Education Program who found themselves encouraged to adopt a normative identity while being groomed as "ambassadors of the profession" (Bourgeault 1996, 129); and immigrant midwives of colour who found themselves largely excluded from practice in the province.

Official norms of antidiscrimination and multiculturalism guarantee that whites do not normally admit to discriminatory practices (van Dijk 1993a). These practices must instead be accessed through the accounts of the racialized minority people who have experienced their impact. "Contrapuntal" methodology shows how the respectability of some midwives has been produced through comparison with a range of "undesirable" midwifery subjects (Said 1993, 52). A critical element of this methodology is the juxtaposition of an analysis of racist exclusion against testimonies about its impact. Such a juxtaposition is also necessary to avoid a self-referential engagement with naming and defining whiteness. If, as Aida Hurtado and Abigail J. Stewart (1997, 308) have observed, "People of Color are experts about whiteness, which we have learned whites most emphatically are not," then these people's testimonies are critical to any attempt to describe how white domination works. Consequently, my analysis draws heavily upon the narratives of twenty-three women of colour, including midwifery students, midwifery board members, and immigrant midwives. Jane Jacobs (1996, 24) acknowledges the risks of presenting and interpreting the words of "those marked as Other in the imperial imagination," admitting that such "intercultural interpretation" is never innocent and that researchers cannot simply divest themselves of their dominant positioning in a "not-so-fraying imperialist world." However, argues Jacobs, an anticolonial project that does *not* take into consideration "how colonialism encounters and is transformed by those it seeks to dominate ... might simply work to embellish the core."

This research brings to the foreground relations of domination and subordination between white women and women of colour, and it does not hesitate to name the perpetuation of white dominance through institutional processes and intersubjective means as racism. Virginia Dominguez (1995, 326) prudently asks "what the invocation of racism accomplishes contextually given a field of available options that range from its silencing to its naming as a different 'thing.'" I would respond that such an invocation is a powerful discursive intervention in modern liberal societies where the irrelevance of race is proclaimed at the same instant that racialized forms of differentiation and exclusion proliferate (Goldberg 1993). Inasmuch as racism today is produced in and through a variety of designations, opinions, exclusions, and rationalizations that appear to have nothing to do with race, we require sophisticated strategies to comprehend its operations. Critical and feminist scholars have not been adequately attentive to these processes, and the installation of race as an indispensable category of analysis in such scholarship is long overdue (Higginbotham 1992; Barbee 1993).

The Writer of the Text

"One learns about method," claims Norman Denzin (1994, 505), "by thinking about how one makes sense of one's own life." In my own case, confrontation with the contradictory aspects of my identity impelled me to pursue the research upon which this text is based and to seek a method that could explain the contradictions that seem to buffet me from one kind of social positioning to another. Thinking back, I remember this process as located in two instructive and emotionally charged moments in which I was rendered first marginal and then dominant in relation to two different groups. The first moment occurred in 1989 when I attended an annual general meeting of the midwives' professional body, the Association of Ontario Midwives (AOM). The second took place in 1995, when more than ten immigrant midwives of colour enrolled in a community college course that I taught. Both of these moments have more than a little to do with my Jewish identity and its relationship to the conditions of forced migration and diaspora in the twentieth century (and now into the twenty-first).

I have been a migrant, albeit an extraordinarily privileged and largely voluntary one. My migrations have been prompted not by touristic longings but by a "dream of belonging" (Pollock 1994, 84) linked to the displacements suffered by previous generations of Jews. In 1988, I came to Canada after having emigrated from the United States to Israel, where I lived for fifteen years. Moving to Israel had been part of my quest for a less fragmented existence. I wanted to live in a place where my cultural and political commitments did not need to be explained and where the rhythms of life and timelines of weekly and yearly rituals and celebrations did not always require negotiation with a Christian majority culture. I wanted to be free to pursue a form of radical left politics that rendered me anathema to the American Jewish community, which increasingly saw "New Left" Jews as a threat to Jewish self-interest and to the respectability and white racial identity – what Karen Brodkin (1998, 39) has called "a whiteness of our own" – claimed by and conferred upon North American Jews in the years following the Second World War (Staub 1999). A peace activist both before and after my emigration to Israel, I eventually gave up hope of a just settlement between Palestinians and Jews. I became tired, as I explained it to those who questioned my reasons for leaving, of being the "master of millions of Arabs," and I left Israel.

In Israel, I had worked as prenatal educator and been involved for many years in a leadership role in the movement for demedicalized, humanized childbearing. In 1989, after returning to Canada, I was in need of work and of a community of activists with whom I could pursue my commitment to childbirth reform. A friend suggested that I get involved in the burgeoning midwifery movement. I recall attending the AOM's annual general meeting that year, and for me, this memory is a visceral one. In a recent autobiographical article, Melanie Kaye/Kantrowitz (1996, 123) compressed all the habits and embodiments that produce gendered Jewish difference in relation to bourgeois white femininity in North America into a moment of physical and emotional intelligence. "Before I knew what a *shiksa* was," confessed Kaye/Kantrowitz, "I knew I wasn't it."[12] On that day in 1989, I also knew I "wasn't it." I recall watching the speakers and feeling the sense of expertise and competence that I had gained in Israel being hopelessly eroded. The women I saw were highly articulate, attractive, and poised. But in my view, they were, above all, characterized by their embodiment of a kind of neutral citizenship. Marks of racial or class difference were absent. These women were precisely the liberal subjects who could make claims to bettering the lot of "women" with no complicated involvements with other categories or designations.

As Caren Kaplan (1998, 453) has argued, white North American Jews frequently experience a cognitive, and not infrequently political, dissonance between our access to privilege and the threat of racism "expressed as antisemitism." For North American Jews in the postwar period, the dissonance produced by multiple and contradictory positioning has frequently been muted through a foregrounding of our claims to subordinate status. We find it difficult, if not impossible, to see the relationship between our successful assimilation (and our whiteness) and our material and discursive relationships to racialized others.[13] As "model immigrants," North American Jews seem to prove liberalism's claim that merit is foremost and race irrelevant in the struggle for social advancement. We embrace this illusion, I believe, because our differentiation from those deemed more paradigmatically human has brought violence upon us again and again. Keeping all this in mind, I want to return to the scene of my own cognitive dissonance – my encounters with immigrant midwives of colour.

In the summer of 1995, the interdisciplinary childbirth educators training program that I had taught for several years – a collaboration between a suburban college and an urban teaching hospital – received nearly triple its usual number of applications for the coming academic year. Even more unusual, half of the students applying were women of colour, most of them trained midwives from countries in the global South. Childbirth education has been an overwhelmingly white avocation in Ontario (and elsewhere in North America), and the opportunity to develop a more diverse pool of childbirth educators was decidedly welcome in a city where "visible minority" people comprise nearly half of the population. However, most of the students of colour came to the program with slightly different intentions. Midwifery had been incorporated into the Ontario health care system in 1994, and many of these women had entered the childbirth educators training program as a way of learning about the alternative birth movement and of preparing for the complex process of becoming registered as midwives through the Prior Learning Assessment program established by the newly formed College of Midwives of Ontario.

Because I moved primarily within white and white-Jewish spaces, had I not encountered this group of women, nothing, not even my own minor sense of marginalization, would have challenged my understanding of the re-emergence of midwifery in Ontario as a laudatory, woman-centred project. Listening to these immigrant women of colour week after week and reading their essays, I was struck by the depth of their knowledge about childbearing, their commitment to humanized maternity care practices, and their clearly feminist positions on issues related to health care. Their integration into the midwifery profession in Ontario should be relatively smooth, I predicted. But as time passed, I realized that I was wrong. I was dismayed to see how, with only one exception, these women retreated from their dream to practise midwifery in Ontario. I, on the other hand, had not been forced to retreat from what I knew best. Shortly after attending the 1989 AOM meeting, I found a job in my field and had found and become involved with advocacy groups in which I felt comfortable. I had no "Canadian experience," but this did not stand in my way. The anomaly represented by these very different outcomes, and the extraordinary ease in integration that my whiteness had purchased, could not be denied. How racialized knowledge was produced and transmitted through romanticizing of "primitive" childbearing practices had been the topic of my recently completed master's thesis, and it was clear to me that issues of race figured powerfully in the midwifery equation as well. I found the need to account for the racialized dimensions of midwifery's re-emergence so compelling that I decided to write this book.

The subordinate aspects of my positioning allow a more critical perception of white dominance, but I am by no means innocent of engaging in its practices nor am I denied most of its privileges. While I can struggle to hear, see, and listen better, my dominance creates epistemological limits. There are, however, as Trinh (1989, 41) notes, "in between grounds" that can be occupied in a struggle to hear/see/listen in ways that acknowledge how power operates in the transmission of knowledge. I have attempted to gain access to these spaces by constantly reassessing how historical legacies and everyday practices restrict what is said and what is heard when I, as a racially dominant woman, research racially subordinate "others." These binary formulations are never secure, and those positioned subordinately exercise authority and subvert dominance in innumerable ways.

Under such conditions, what kinds of claims can be made and what can they be expected to achieve? I have consciously composed a new tale in which I unravel the strands of Ontario midwifery's "heroic" story and introduce newly collected threads spun from previously unheard narratives and disparate statistics, documents, and theories, reweaving them into an alternative telling. This new telling of the story of the re-emergence of midwifery in the province reverses the heroic fable of women's gain to show its underside of racial dominance. While such a reweaving is primarily a discursive intervention, shifts in discourse necessarily precede material shifts in power. "As alternative stories become available," explains Jane Flax (1998, 10), "more subjects are likely to resist." For white women involved in midwifery and other feminist projects, the counternarrative that I have constructed might provide a road map for thinking beyond the dominant positions into which we have been structured. We cannot transcend those positionings, but we can certainly begin to learn how to avoid reproducing dominance from within them, and we can and must struggle to reconstruct the institutions that perpetuate our dominance. For those who have already begun to address midwifery's history of exclusion, I provide ample empirical evidence with which they can argue that what has been dismissed by those in power as an unfounded or exaggerated claim is, in fact, an inequity that requires redress.[14]

Having devoted more than a decade to the reform of medicalized childbirth and the expansion of childbearing options for women, I have struggled greatly with my own "betrayal" of the midwifery project. My traitorous stance was brought home to me after my first public talk about the research. A midwifery student with whom I was friendly called to ask whether "they" (meaning the midwifery educators in the province's Midwifery Education Program who had attacked my research) were "burning crosses" on my lawn.[15] The imagery of racist and anti-Jewish violence that framed the student's question jarred me, but I don't believe that she chose her words carelessly. Images of burning crosses captured for her the intensity of the opposition she had witnessed. It is my guess that such a response reflects the deep resistance that white women have to acknowledging the limits of our own innocence and the resistance we mount to viewing charges of racism as something more than the biased or hypersensitive imaginings of people of colour and antiracist whites (Essed 1991, 272). While these resistant responses have both troubled and frightened me, I have not been immune to experiencing them myself. They have surfaced as nagging doubts about the veracity of seemingly incontrovertible facts and incontestable interview data that I gathered about the exclusions suffered by racialized minority women. I needed constant reassurance that my claims were not exaggerated, and that what I was describing was indeed racism and not some other phenomenon. While this doubt has driven me to be exceedingly cautious in my claims, it has also forced me to confront how deeply committed we who enjoy race privilege are to versions of racism that allow us to refuse being implicated in the racialized order of things.

Collecting the Data

My positioning as a politically engaged researcher with a history as a childbirth reform activist and antiracist educator worked both for and against me as I gathered documents and conducted the interviews with forty-seven women that helped to shape this book.[16] My past activism and work as a childbirth educator facilitated access to five white midwives whom I define as "nonelite."[17] These women, who knew me or knew of me, agreed eagerly to be interviewed because they viewed my research as a venue for articulating their dissatisfaction with the way midwifery had been integrated into the health care system in Ontario. My work as the coordinator of a childbirth educator program was also key in negotiating interviews with white members of midwifery boards, midwifery students, and immigrant midwives of colour. Many of my former students who had been accepted to the province's Midwifery Education Program had maintained contact with me, and they related their experiences in the program, often with a critical attention to power dynamics. I even received two e-mail requests from students asking to participate in the research, which they saw as important in the struggle to diversify the profession.

Booking and conducting interviews with immigrant midwives of colour and with some of the few women of colour who participated on midwifery boards posed different challenges. Some of the interviews were conducted with students or colleagues with whom I shared a concern about the exclusion of women of colour from midwifery. The interviews with these women were easy to negotiate. The remaining interviews with immigrant midwives of colour were largely brokered for me by this first group of women.[18] In most cases, their "recommendations" of me opened a door that might otherwise have been closed.[19] However, the recommendation did not always yield an immediate agreement to meet. One woman expressed interest in being interviewed and told me she had a "big story" to tell. She also expressed concern that she might jeopardize herself by agreeing to be interviewed. We spent an hour on the telephone discussing the various ways in which her identity could be disguised (neither her name, nor names of colleagues or institutions where she worked, would be used; no country of origin would accompany her quotes; if she wished, she could see how I had contextualized the quotes).[20] She told me to call back in a month. I sent her a copy of a paper I had written on racist exclusion in the Ontario midwifery movement and a letter introducing the research (see Appendix A). By the time of the next call, she had had some extremely negative experiences with a midwifery practice and agreed eagerly to the interview. With other potential interview subjects, I followed the same sequence of sending the paper and the introductory letter after I had made initial phone contact. I believe that my having established myself as a critic of midwifery's exclusionary policies, rather than as a neutral researcher, is what gained me interviews with some white students and with most women of colour.[21] All participants were sent transcripts of the interviews and were invited to change, excise, or add material, which about half did. Most made corrections to their grammar or crossed out the names of institutions that they had mentioned.[22] However, some women felt that they had told me more than was safe to tell. Two women called me to express their hesitation around having their words made public. They felt that they might be identified or, in one case, held liable for breaching a non-disclosure agreement. In each case, the women chose to stay in the study but laid down specific conditions about how the information was to be used. In one case, I agreed to send a woman the exact text where her quote appeared and asked that she relay her approval by phone before I submitted the chapter of the manuscript containing her quote for publication.

My reputation as a critic definitely gained me interviews with those who had experienced exclusion or those who opposed it, but it blocked my access to midwifery's elite.[23] Although I had decided to limit the number of interviews with key midwifery activists, I felt obligated to hear how at least a few of them explained the scarcity of women of colour in the profession. I was reluctant to make these contacts, inasmuch as friends and former students had told me in what disparaging terms my work had been discussed by two of the three women I hoped to interview. I waited until late in the study to attempt these interviews, as I wanted to feel completely sure about the claims I was making. Only one woman agreed to talk to me. Early on in our interview, I abandoned my list of questions because her responses were so intractably embedded in a heroic tale of midwifery and in an unreflective analytical frame that it seemed absurd to proceed. She was simply recounting the official story that I had read in a hundred versions before arriving in her office. I also contacted two women who occupied key roles in the midwifery bureaucracy and the education program. I left telephone messages for these women on three occasions, then sent each a letter and one an e-mail message. Approximately seven weeks later one of the women responded, but she refused an interview and offered a letter instead. I was not surprised by these (non)responses; rather they confirmed to me that to preserve midwifery's coherent identity as progressive, feminist, and moral, criticism could be neither tolerated nor abetted.

I have not occupied the role of distanced and "objective" researcher in this project. My anxieties, both potential and real, have shaped these pages in innumerable ways. I have wrestled daily with the fear that I might betray the women of colour whom I have interviewed by misrepresenting them or representing them so well that they could be recognized. They reminded me over and over again, through the process of negotiating the conditions of the research, that I must assume responsibility for mitigating the risk that they took by agreeing to be interviewed. I hope that I have accomplished this task adequately.

Overview

Chapters 1 and 2 form a detailed and chronological documentation of the way racist exclusion has worked in the Ontario midwifery project. From the outset, the very terms of self-definition that midwives developed and deployed precluded the participation of immigrant midwives of colour. Attempts at including the voices of marginalized groups in the midwifery project predominantly served to secure rather than to undo white dominance. In chapter 3, I detail how the mobility of some midwives within the health care system has been linked to having access to birthing mothers in the Third World. Ontario midwives were transformed into more respectable health care professionals by having travelled to midwifery clinics in Third World countries where they could gain status and expertise not available to them at home.[24] Chapter 4 looks at the construction of a normative midwifery subject and tracks how white midwives who threatened midwifery respectability were either purged or transformed through a set of disciplinary practices that continue to be applied to students entering the Midwifery Education Program. In chapter 5, I examine how midwives of colour have been regulated by racist exclusion, and I document their descriptions of and responses to this process. In the Conclusion, I consider my own accountability to the women of colour who were my research subjects, and I ponder both the liberatory potential of a racially inclusive midwifery profession and the limitations of feminist resistance conceptualized and deployed from within racist structures.

1
Technologies of Exclusion

> White women can no longer see ourselves as innocent of the domination of others due to our oppression by men. If for no other reason, this realization should make race a matter of urgency for all those interested in gendering.
>
> – Jane Flax, *Disputed Subjects*

The movement to legalize midwifery in Ontario is a cogent example of the potential pitfalls of projects intended to address "the universal needs of women" (Glenn 1992, 37). Feminist projects that posit a shared female identity across categories of difference and that fail to take into account how women are positioned as both dominant and subordinate in relation to one another are themselves fated to reproduce relations of domination. Epistemological frameworks that see gender as a discrete category and not as one produced in and through other dimensions of social identity such as class, sexuality, and race ignore differences between women. Unable to see past their own sense of oppression, midwifery activists chose a political route that sustained rather than challenged systems that marginalized other women. Racial segmentation in the nursing labour force, the deskilling of immigrant workers, and derogatory and retrograde representations of women of colour are but a few of the systems the Ontario midwifery movement relied upon in its bid to challenge a patriarchal maternity care system. It is not a surprise that the benefits of this movement have not accrued universally to all women but rather to a highly circumscribed elite.

The achievement of legalized midwifery must be viewed in relation to both discursive and material processes in which Third World women, including those displaced to the North by oppressive transnational economic policies, have played significant roles. Conceptually, images of Third World women have served to define middle-class white women's midwifery identities through both negative comparison *and* fantasized idealization. In decidedly material ways, flesh and blood Third World women, within the health care system and elsewhere in the economy, buttress dominant female positions, including those of white midwives. In addition, Third World women have frequently provided the clinical experience that Ontario midwives who travelled to the South later traded for professional status.

By tracing the identity categories into which those excluded from midwifery are structured, we can bring the interrelationship of race, class, and gender into view. The disqualification of many, if not most, midwives of colour represents a discrete dimension of the re-emergence of midwifery in Ontario. Nurses, rural women, counterculture women, and women who have not attended institutions of higher education have been subject to exclusionary treatment as well. The proximity of these identity categories to the discourses of "degeneracy" is significant. The necessity of constructing boundaries between "degenerate" female subjects and white middle-class ones was fundamental in the process that established Canada's first registered midwives.

Building the Technologies of Exclusion:
Domestic Workers and Nurses

The migration of Third World women to developed countries, and their engagement here in what has been historically understood as "women's work," have been long-overdue subjects of scholarly investigation (Ehrenreich and Hochschild 2002; Parreñas 2001). Indeed, feminist scholars are only just beginning to theorize the ways in which migrant women, working both as domestic labourers and in traditionally female professions such as nursing, enable the occupational mobility of some First World women. Canadian scholars Abigail Bakan and Daiva Stasiulis have demonstrated, in concrete terms, how systems of subordination interlock in the case of foreign domestic workers in Canada (Bakan and Stasiulis 1995, 1997; Stasiulis and Bakan 2003). They describe how a need for child care in dual-income middle-class families comes to be filled by female migrant workers from Third World countries. The "suitability" of these women to household labour, a key ideological component of the process that Bakan and Stasiulis (1995, 305) describe, is linked to the role of domestic placement agencies in reproducing "a highly racialized set of practices and criteria in the recruitment and placement of female non-citizen domestic workers in Canadian households." Demonstrating the link between discursive and material practices, Bakan and Stasiulis (1995) have shown that the decline in the number of domestic workers entering Canada from the Caribbean under the Live-in Caregiver Program and the concomitant rise in entrants from the Philippines are directly linked to racist stereotyping by domestic placement agencies.[1] While the agency owners (and potential employers) differentiate between Filipino and Afro-Caribbean applicants in equally racist ways, they have used racist discourses about Afro-Caribbean applicants that have produced these women as unsuitable for employment as domestic workers. Such pernicious discourses, which have long antecedents, have arisen simultaneously with organized resistance on the part of Afro-Caribbean domestic workers to inhuman conditions of employment and unfair immigration practices.

The work of Bakan and Stasiulis demonstrates the complicity of middle-class Canadian women in the oppression of Third World women. The employment of migrant women as domestic workers enables some modification of the gender division of labour because it facilitates white women's participation in the labour force. However, this transformation of the gendered division of labour leaves the racial division of labour unchanged. An array of systems continues to connect women in ways that are both "hierarchical and interdependent" (Glenn 1992, 37). Creating child care solutions that do not demand hierarchical relations between women would require a reconfiguration of all the systems described above.

Feminist work on the topic of foreign domestic labour also illustrates how "the international is personal" (Enloe 1989, 196). That some white women's occupational mobility has been enabled by the social reproductive labour of women from Third World countries, who undertake for them such domestic tasks such as cooking, laundry, and child care, has been increasingly acknowledged by feminist scholars.[2] The case of foreign domestic workers, however, is only one example of the ways in which global processes interact with local ones to produce a local labour force stratified by gender, race, class, and access to citizenship rights. The intense focus on foreign domestic labour has been of critical importance. This focus now needs to be widened so that we can account for the ways in which the same dynamics have operated within other sectors, including the health care labour force, in which nursing is becoming an increasingly globalized commodity (Kofman 2004).

Professional nursing in the industrialized West constitutes a particularly dense site of meaning-making in relation to race, class, and gender. As this young woman, a first-year student at prestigious Wellesley College, demonstrates, gender requires race and class for its intelligibility: "If I were to say I wanted to become a nurse ... my professors and fellow students would think that I was crazy. To them, it would be like saying I wanted to be a janitor" (Gordon 1991, 124). Here, nursing, seen as a subservient form of female employment and one unsuited to middle-class women who have more attractive occupational options, is coded by race through the speaker's references to janitorial work, a job frequently done in the United States and Canada by racial-minority workers and immigrant people of colour. It is by negative reference to an array of degraded/degenerate identities structured in and through class, race, and gender that a middle-class white female identity emerges.

Degeneracy, in its emergent form as a pathologizing discourse of nineteenth-century medicine, was used to "sharpen the distinction between normal and abnormal, between the bourgeois virtues which led to progress and the vices which led to the extinction of the individual, the family, and the national community" (Mosse 1985, 35). "Degenerate classes" are no less necessary to the creation of social boundaries and to the definition of the white bourgeois subject today than they were then. Stoler (1995,15) argues that "civilities and social hygiene" were of primary importance in creating the healthy bodies of the white bourgeoisie and that these criteria were always "measured in racial terms." The production of contemporary middle-class identities is evident in the recent construction of a new elite configuration of nursing professionals. "Civilities and social hygiene," always embedded in a matrix of racial meanings, are invoked in the process of securing middle-class female identities within an increasingly proletarian and racialized nursing profession.

Racial segmentation is a prominent feature of nursing in both Canada and the United States. The majority of highly skilled nursing labour is performed by white registered nurses. Lower-skilled nursing and caretaking tasks are performed by licensed practical nurses, nurses' aides, and home care workers; significant numbers of these are women of colour (Stasiulis and Bakan 2003); Calliste 1996). The recent thrust to create a nursing elite constructs a defining border between the working-class aspects of nursing labour and its more scientific and intellectual ones. By claiming a unique body of scientific nursing knowledge, elite nurses are seeking to assume more of the curative labour traditionally performed by physicians (Carpenter 1993). Managerial expertise and scientific knowledge secured through elite education characterize the move to reconfigure nursing practice and distance it from its proletarian underpinnings.[3] Nursing elites depend on a "toehold on respectability" (Fellows and Razack 1998) to distinguish themselves from subordinates.

Among the entire range of dividing discourses that distinguish respectable bodies from degenerate ones, now, as in the nineteenth century, "cultural competencies, sexual proclivities, psychological dispositions, and cultivated habits" (Stoler 1995, 141) position variously embodied subjects within a shifting matrix of respectability. Social boundaries continue to be configured along lines that can be traced back to nineteenth-century discourses of degeneracy in which "healthy" nations distanced themselves from those who imperilled normative identities.

These boundaries are drawn between those with university training and those whose education is acquired in more accessible and less prestigious institutions like community colleges; between labour in which traditional female caring skills are the major component and labour that is more medical and managerial; between work that involves significant contact with dirt and human effluvia and work that is relatively clean. The outlines of degenerate identities from a previous era are detectable, and they emerge along the intersecting lines of class (manual versus mental labour) and gender (servile versus resistant womanhood), in which the subordinate positioning in each couplet has a racially based referent in society. In Canada, such borders are also drawn along the highly racialized lines of citizen/ noncitizen, inasmuch as foreign-trained professionals, including nurses, frequently have great difficulty in having their credentials recognized (Ontario 2002).[4] Transnational processes have had an unmistakable impact on the health care labour force in Canada. The massive debt load of former colonies to financial institutions like the World Bank, and the structural adjustment policies demanded by these institutions, have produced an economic upheaval in which masses of migrant workers, including highly skilled ones such as immigrant midwives/nurses of colour, seek a living outside of their home countries in the South.[5] The decisions of medical workers to migrate, however, cannot be seen simply as the "free-choice" prerogative of an occupational elite. The migration of doctors, nurses, midwives, and other health care professionals to First World countries must be viewed as part of a global movement of migrants seeking employment. The number of these migrants has reached nearly 200 million (United Nations 2003). The movement of medical workers takes place in a very specific economic context in which benefits accrue to First World receiver countries, further degrading the living conditions of most residents of Third World sender countries.[6]

Some feminist theorists insist that the gender division in health care mirrors "the traditional division of labor between men and women in the family" (Butter et al. 1987, 140), with women responsible for such tasks as cleaning, education, caring, counselling, and so on, and men accountable for the more prestigious and intellectually demanding "curative" work. I contend that the health care labour force resembles not the "traditional" family but the newly reconstituted bourgeois family in which migrant and immigrant women of colour and other marginalized women perform the fundamental caring duties, allowing the (white, middle-class) woman of the family to pursue more prestigious, lucrative, and autonomous forms of work.[7] Such a claim must be considered in relation to the inability of Canadian nursing schools to meet the demands for nursing personnel (Ross-Kerr and Wood 2002, 23), the overrepresentation of immigrant women of colour in the health care labour force (Preston and Giles 1997), and their lack of representation proportional to their numbers in managerial positions in nursing (Stasiulis and Bakan 2003, 129; Calliste 2000, 150; Caissey 1994). What must also be taken into consideration is the streaming of nurses of colour into low-status units such as chronic care, rehabilitation, and geriatrics, where advancement is unlikely and occupational injury more common (Caissey 1994; Lum and Williams 2000).[8]

As provincial and federal budget cuts shift health care from institutions to the home, women increasingly experience the burden as unpaid labour. While this unequal burden reflects a gendered division of labour, it is also unequally distributed across class and race boundaries (Glazer 1988). Those who can afford to do so will hire registered nurses, nursing assistants, or home aides to perform work created through this policy. Immigrant nurses who are prevented from becoming registered (because they lack English proficiency, and/or resources to prepare for and pay for licensing examinations, and so on) may come to perform these jobs in unregulated and/or non-unionized workplaces where conditions and remuneration are substandard. The interlocking relations of domination with regard to hierarchies of class, race, and gender are clearly visible in the recent health care crisis in Canada.

Midwifery: The Chronology of Exclusion

Prelegislation Midwifery as a White Space

The re-emergence of midwifery in the 1970s in Ontario represents a convergence of multiple and sometimes conflicting forces, including feminist and traditional women's health movements (including those which challenged the medical management of childbirth); counterculture lifestyle practices; and efforts by largely British-trained midwives to have their skills recognized within the health care system.[9] The revival of home birth, which had been systematically eradicated in Canada and the United States by the mid-twentieth century, played a key role in midwifery's revival.[10] In the 1960s and early 1970s, some women from Ontario's largest city, Toronto, including some from marginalized religious communities, and others who, with their partners, sought birth experiences outside of the hospital setting, used the services of doctors willing to provide care at home births (Bourgeault 1996, 37). In 1976, funding cuts to the Victorian Order of Nurses (VON) meant that home-birth doctors lost access to formally trained assistants, and that their clients forfeited follow-up care by nurses in the immediate postpartum period. The Home Birth Task Force, organized to lobby for restoration of VON services, became the springboard for the development of community-based midwifery training, and ultimately for the movement to integrate midwifery into Ontario's health care system.

In the next decade, two groups followed quite different trajectories in their quests to give Ontario residents access to midwifery care. Some foreign-trained nurse-midwives, primarily white women from Britain, had formed the Ontario Nurse-Midwives Association (ONMA) in September of 1973 (Ontario Nurse-Midwives Association n.d.). The group went on to gather information and lobby medical and nursing organizations for the incorporation of some form of midwifery care into the health care system. Many were labour and delivery nurses working in hospitals, and they assiduously avoided participating in out-of-hospital deliveries for fear of losing their nursing credentials and/or their jobs (Bourgeault 1996, 43). It was not until 1981 that the ONMA connected with the recently formed Ontario Association of Midwives (OAM), a support group consisting of women who were working as birth assistants and midwives, and parents and others who supported midwifery. An outgrowth of the Home Birth Task Force, the group boasted nearly two hundred members by 1982 (Bourgeault 1996, 39). Eleanor Barrington (1985, 16), a chronicler of midwifery, writes that "by 1980, the majority of midwives and their clients belonged to the middle class. Today's 'wise woman' is likely to be about thirty-five, raised in a suburb and university educated." Arguably, most of Barrington's descriptives are code words for white racial identity. That the early midwifery movement was, almost without exception, composed of white women is accepted as fact by the veteran midwives and midwifery activists interviewed in the course of this research.[11]

Only three of the five white veteran midwives interviewed, all of whom have been active in midwifery since the mid-1970s and are currently practising, were able to recall the presence of women of colour during the earliest years of the movement.[12] Two mentioned the same practitioner, a woman who attempted to become registered in the province but who ultimately withdrew. One Toronto midwife remembered that a colleague in another city had worked with "a black woman who had been a midwife somewhere else, and I remember I met that woman just once" (Interview no. 19). In a few cases, when asked to recall women of colour who became involved in midwifery, interviewees mentioned women who might be described as "white others" – not quite proficient in the cultural competencies that would allow them to merge easily into midwifery's mainstream, but also unlikely to be identified as visible minority people in a system of racial differentiation in which skin colour is the primary reference point.

One interview subject remembered an Italian midwife who regularly attended OAM meetings but eventually stopped coming. Recalled another veteran midwife, "One of them who was practising was ... Argentinean, and she had also practised in Holland and in Israel, and she spoke like five languages ... And she actually became quite involved and she got into our circles" (Interview no. 17). Yet another veteran white midwife remembered that "there was one woman who came here from Holland. That was in the '80s. She wasn't black but she ... was a practising midwife in Holland" (Interview no. 19). Such responses, I believe, indicate how unusual it was to encounter women who differed in any way from Barrington's description of midwives quoted above. One veteran midwife who admitted that she remembered no one who was not white, educated, and middle class quipped, "The most diverse was people coming from the United States!" (Interview no. 21).

Spaces of Encounter

Ontario midwives and immigrant midwives of colour *did*, however, encounter one another, and these encounters occurred most frequently in contexts with especially strong links to gender and globalization: health care and child care. White midwives frequently accompanied their clients to the hospital, where they were prevented from engaging in clinical care but could provide needed emotional and physical support to the labouring woman. In such a setting, they met and interacted in the prelegislation period with midwives of colour who worked as labour and delivery nurses. In Toronto, where more than one-third of nurses are immigrant women of colour, these encounters would have been almost impossible to avoid. One white midwife admitted that she just as frequently encountered immigrant midwives of colour working as nannies for her clients as she did nurses in hospitals. Describing her interaction with these women, this veteran midwife said, "Sometimes, I would say, [they] were very friendly and sort of said, 'I was a midwife from my own country, you know!' and there was a very collegial feeling about that ... We talked just experiences kind of thing. But sometimes women would say ... I've been asked like, 'who do you contact [to become a midwife in Ontario] ?' and whatever" (Interview no. 20).

These postcolonial spaces of encounter structure the stories that can be told about the women who inhabit them (Grewal 1996). In the prelegislation period, white midwives and immigrant midwives of colour were employed in the health care system in subordinate and non-commensurate ways. Midwives of colour working as labour and delivery nurses were subordinate to doctors and frequently to white nurses; however, they also commanded institutional authority in relation to prelegislation midwives, whose presence in the hospital as labour support was met with varying levels of enthusiasm among staff. White midwives may have been looked upon with suspicion and disdain by both doctors and nurses, who resented their supposed antimedical stance and claim to expert knowledge, but the women's white, middle-class identity may also have afforded some advantages.

Alone among those interviewed, one midwife frequently directed midwives of colour to the various routes to professional practice available to them and has a long record of resistance to exclusionary policies. Encounters between white midwives and immigrant midwives of colour described in other interviews never involved the exchange of information that might encourage the non-practising midwives to become involved in midwifery-related activities. One immigrant midwife of colour who was among the small handful who participated in prelegislation midwifery activities recalls that her own training and aspirations to practise, as well as the constraints on her ability to do so, were largely ignored by the white midwives she encountered, some of whom later became key policy makers:

> I think I expressed interest certainly, ultimately that I'd like to practise but because of my status, I didn't want to practise in the way that they were practising currently, because I was just afraid about earning an income and not having my status. I was only allowed to work ... I was only supposed to work as a babysitter. But it was so tenuous as well, and because I really wanted to stay in Canada I didn't want to do anything to jeopardize it ... I don't recall anybody saying, "I want you to come to a birth with me and see how you feel, see if you really want to." People knew, they knew that I really passionately wanted to do midwifery here ... It just occurred to me, there was never anything. (Interview no. 6)

Four out of the five midwives of colour interviewed who had worked as labour and delivery nurses before the legalization of midwifery recalled meeting white midwives in the hospital setting. Two of these women remembered that colleagues regarded the midwives with suspicion, seeing legalization as a potential threat to nursing jobs. However, one did remember the interaction as pleasant and collegial. "We had a delivery, quite nice. So we kind of appreciated them, and then they said, 'Oh, you guys are doing quite well too.' We kind of appreciated each other, and then we said, 'The mechanics of birth are always the same' ... They did want to know who we are. And then we did want to know who they are, too" (Interview no. 2). Interactions between midwives of colour working as labour and delivery nurses and white midwives in the prelegislation period were varied, ranging from indifference and hostility to enthusiastic support.

There were other settings in which these groups met. One white midwife described how she invited foreign-trained midwives, including women of colour, to share their skills at in-service seminars. Because they were not practising midwives, these women were barred, later in the seminar, from attending the peer-review session of local midwives that was part of the self-regulatory process in the years before legislation. "I think they felt quite eliminated when they weren't allowed to be in on those meetings, the veteran midwife told me" (Interview no. 16).

Why would these two groups not have found enough common ground to forge personal and political links? From the point of view of midwifery activists, it can be argued that a number of discourses, including inferiorization of nurses, their construction as subservient to doctors, and their assumed acquiescence to conventional medicine, converged with racist discourses, including those about Third World medical training, to produce a subject wholly antithetical to the respectable, feminist subject the midwifery movement was struggling to construct. For midwives of colour working as labour and delivery nurses, their own claims to special professional knowledge were undermined by the presence in the workplace of these white and, for the most part, empirically trained midwives. The immigrant midwives of colour who were interviewed used a variety of discursive strategies to retain their status as midwives despite being prevented by midwifery legislation from claiming that title. Immigrant midwives of colour struggling to achieve professional status and workplace security as nurses might have logically desired to maintain their distance from a midwifery movement seen to represent counterculture and antimedical values.

While interactions between immigrant midwives of colour and white midwives were relatively infrequent and took place under circumstances characterized by complexity, they did occur. In some spaces, these groups were structured into the system in ways that virtually guaranteed that they would not seek common ground. Still, there were numerous opportunities to explore points of professional convergence. Consequently, exclusionary policies and attitudes were enacted not from a racially bounded space of ignorance, but from a position of knowledge, however limited, of the skills and aspirations of the women with whom white midwives came into contact in the prelegislation period.

Few midwives of colour participated in prelegislation midwifery, nor did the midwifery movement constitute a diverse environment in terms of clientele. Veteran white midwives whom I interviewed, all of whom had extremely active practices (thirty to forty births a year as primary care provider) in urban settings, had slightly different but uniformly low estimates of the number of women of colour they served in the years before legalized midwifery. One veteran reported that she had "about forty births in a year [...] Out of those, a couple would not be, would not be ... white people" (Interview no. 20). Another midwife estimated the number to be "one percent?, if [that]" (Interview no. 19). One of the few immigrant midwives of colour to practise in the pre-legislation period indicated that the bulk of her clientele was white, with clients of colour accounting for "maybe 5 percent, actually" (Interview no. 17). Asked why she thought that women from her own immigrant community did not seek midwifery care, she replied that she felt that the cost of care had been a deterrent to potential clients and that she herself couldn't afford to do as many "free births" as she would have liked (Interview no. 17).

The Outreach Committee of the Association of Ontario Midwives, 1984-93

Immigrant midwives of colour had little to do with the midwifery revival in the province other than as imagined partners. Used in this role they constituted a useful bargaining chip in convincing the provincial government of the need for midwives. In 1983, the province began a review of health professions, with the global aim of revamping how these professions were regulated in Ontario.[13] The Health Professions Legislation Review (HPLR) contacted numerous organizations, among them the Ontario Association of Midwives (OAM) and the Ontario Nurse-Midwives Association (ONMA), to ascertain whether midwifery should be regulated as a health profession (Bourgeault 1996, 42). The HPLR proved to be a pivotal event in the re-emergence of midwifery, as midwives and their supporters began to direct substantial effort toward being incorporated into Ontario's health care system. The OAM and the ONMA joined with the Midwifery Task Force of Ontario (MTFO), a newly formed consumer support group, to produce a brief for presentation to the HPLR.[14] With the turn toward legalization came what appears to be the first public statement about access by marginalized groups to midwifery care and practice. Unlike the equity positions articulated by midwifery bodies in subsequent years, this statement acknowledged that the access to care by marginalized groups and their access to midwifery practice were interrelated. It named the material resources that the achievement of equity between dominant and marginalized groups required: "Given the substantial benefits that accrue to lower-class and immigrant women through midwifery care, it seems clear that midwives would be recruited and educated from as broad an ethnic and class range as possible. Access to midwifery education then, for those who might otherwise be excluded, should be guaranteed by means of subsidized training programs; in northern regions of Canada, such programs should be particularly geared to the training of Native women" (Midwifery Task Force of Ontario 1984, 7). Notwithstanding unsubstantiated claims about midwifery's benefits to "lower-class and immigrant women" and the racializing effects of this form of representation, this is perhaps the most progressive and inclusive statement to appear in midwifery publications. As legalization approached, concerns with equity grew less radical, less urgent, and far less pragmatic.

In November of 1984 the OAM and ONMA agreed to merge, creating the Association of Ontario Midwives (AOM n.d., 1). One of the AOM's goals, stated in the first issue of its newsletter, was "outreach – to include the many midwives unable to practise their profession in Ontario," among them those trained outside of Canada (AOM n.d., 4). On the agenda for the group's first annual general meeting was the establishment of an "outreach committee." Other AOM committees, such as the legislative and professional advisory committees, published reports in the organization's newsletter. Reports from the outreach committee were absent from the publication in the organization's first few years. The issue of foreign-trained midwives, however, did concern the AOM. How midwives would be educated and integrated into the health care system become a pressing matter in 1985. In that year, a coroner's inquest investigating the death of a baby whose mother was attended by midwives recommended the regulation of midwifery in the province. This outcome influenced a similar recommendation by the HPLR and led ultimately to the legislature admitting midwives to practice on 31 December 1993 (Bourgeault 1996, 70).

In their 1985 submission to the HPLR, the AOM outlined its plan for the integration of midwifery into the health care system in Ontario. It recommended that "only midwives who have attended a minimum of 50 births, 30 of them as primary caregivers, be considered. These midwives must have been trained and/or [have] practised in the last five years either in Ontario or in a foreign jurisdiction" (MTFO 1986, 11). The AOM's plan for legalized midwifery stipulated that foreign-trained midwives who had graduated from accredited schools and who had trained in the previous five years needed only to provide evidence of their certification to be eligible for a phased-in training program. The policy relating to foreign-trained midwives underwent significant revision as midwifery moved closer to integration into the health care system. Ultimately it prevented many immigrant midwives, among them numerous women of colour, from re-entering their profession with the advent of legalization.

In 1987, the AOM board was concerned with reviving the inactive outreach committee, and a motion was unanimously passed designating the committee's main priority to be "the needs and concerns of rural midwives" (AOM 1987a, 12). This motion was soon amended to include "minority group midwives, at this time particularly, the Inuit" (AOM 1987b, 9). In the period prior to legislation, the AOM seemed to invest time and resources in forging links with a variety of "traditional midwives." Its Fall 1987 newsletter reports at length upon the travels of outreach committee chair Betty-Anne Putt to Canada's North to meet with traditional midwives, as well as to Nicaragua and to various international conferences (AOM 1987a, 10). The newsletter devotes nearly two full pages to these events, as well as to a discussion of Putt's efforts to establish sites abroad where Ontario midwives could gain clinical experience, such as in Sierra Leone, Algeria, the Dutch Antilles, and Malaysia.

Strong in their belief that the instinctual birth behaviours of Western women had been perilously eroded, some Ontario midwives saw themselves as the First World guardians of traditional birthing knowledge, the richest repository of which was thought to exist among Third World midwives. Interactions such as Putt's with Third World midwives – and widespread "midwifery tourism" – conferred a significant degree of midwifery authenticity upon Ontario midwives in their quest for validation. Far from benign, these interactions represent a form of imperialism wherein, as bell hooks (1992, 25) has argued, "the suffering imposed by structures of domination on those designated Other is deflected by an emphasis on seduction and longing where the desire is not to make the Other over in one's image but to become the

Other." This longing for the "other" had its limitations inasmuch as the midwife who is desired is the mythical purveyor of unmediated birthing knowledge encountered in situ, not the fully historicized migrant midwife transported to the First World by conditions of globalization.

A short paragraph inserted into the report of Putt's activities hints, however, at some fleeting awareness on the part of the AOM of the contradiction posed by pursuing the traditional midwife into her Third World habitat when the Third World already has an undeniable presence in the First World. "It will be an important project," reported the AOM newsletter, "to contact all the midwives in Ontario who have been trained in other countries as midwives to help them to become incorporated into the new health care system. This has to be discussed" (AOM 1987b, 10). In a tacit recognition of the predominance of immigrant midwives of colour among those who might wish to become registered, the outreach committee recommended that ads be placed in "ethnic" newspapers, a suggestion that was followed in Eastern Ontario, but not in Toronto, where the visible-minority immigrant population was far greater.

Throughout 1988, reports of the outreach committee in the AOM newsletter dealt exclusively with Betty-Anne Putt's travels and connections with traditional midwives. Sparse news followed in 1989. One midwifery activist told me that the committee was disbanded in that year under circumstances that she was prevented from describing to me by a vow of institutional confidentiality (Interview no. 17). The paralysis that afflicted the outreach committee was multifaceted. First, it never attracted the most politically influential members of the midwifery movement. Second, there was a lingering tension among midwives and their supporters between those who defended regulation and those who regarded it with suspicion.[15] Third, as AOM members were increasingly called upon to serve on provincial boards and committees related to midwifery legislation and implementation, those with political and organizational skills were catapulted into positions of power and influence. Many of the most active were members of the Midwives Collective, a feminist-identified group that paid its members to do political in addition to clinical midwifery work, and whose members seemed to have fewer domestic responsibilities than other practitioners (Bourgeault 1996, 46). The outreach committee rapidly became a refuge for those who were excluded from public midwifery work due to their purported lack of political acumen, their opposition to incorporation, their geographic isolation, or their inability (largely owing to child rearing responsibilities) to devote time to both midwifery politics and midwifery practice. One veteran midwife claimed that the committee "became this place ... it was like a haven for people to come and join with each other and share ideas about what was going on around the province. It became a haven for the rural midwives, it became a place where they felt safe. It became a place where they could talk about what they really wanted to talk about. And at one point, it became a place where people joined if they had different ideologies and were really concerned about legislation and were more interested in decriminalization" (Interview no. 17).

In 1990, the outreach committee, now under the leadership of Teresa Maloney, proposed yet another mandate: "(1) to make contact and promote exchange between the AOM and midwives and students in Ontario who are isolated by such factors as geography, ethnic origin, or need for support; (2) to provide information about the AOM and encourage involvement and; (3) to work toward equal access to midwifery education and to midwifery care for all those who may be discriminated against on the basis of such factors as language, culture, age, economic status, sexual orientation, gender, geographic location, disability, race or religion" (AOM 1990, 13). This was a much more aggressive and comprehensive equity agenda than any that had preceded it. At the same time, an equity committee was established within the Interim Regulatory Council on Midwifery, the body that had been appointed by the provincial government to integrate midwifery into the health care system. The outreach committee of the AOM was never an effective body and it became even less functional in the years just prior to legalization, meeting only once a year (AOM 1991, 20). In 1992, the struggling committee was again restructured so that regions could implement their own outreach projects, although no outreach activities are described in the regional reports in the *AOM 1991/1992 Report*. The report does state, however, that in 1993 the mandate for an outreach/equity committee was being drawn up (AOM 1993, 16).

The outreach committee, the AOM's appointed body for dealing with marginalized midwifery groups, was itself marginal within an organization increasingly concerned with drafting policies that would serve those already practising in the province. Internal fragmentation was not the only factor contributing to the committee's inertia; there were also compelling conceptual and strategic reasons to neglect the outreach issue. Inasmuch as midwives saw themselves as unfairly and rigorously marginalized, an effort to include racialized midwives may well have been a low priority. Inclusivity may have been seen as a liability to a movement clamouring for respectability.

Government Bodies and Exclusionary Policies during the Integration Period

In 1986, the provincial government accepted the Health Professions Legislation Review's recommendation that midwifery become a regulated profession and established the Task Force on the Implementation of Midwifery in Ontario (TFIMO). The task force's mandate was to supply the minister of health with information on midwifery education, scope of practice, governance, and a variety of other matters (TFIMO 1987, 29). Chaired by prominent feminist lawyer Mary Eberts, the task force included a physician, a Canadian nursing professor trained as a nurse-midwife in the United States, and the chair of the Health Professions Legislation Review. Even though no midwives sat on the body, they did exercise considerable influence over its proceedings. The Association of Ontario Midwives and its closely allied support group, the Midwifery Task Force of Ontario, organized numerous submissions to the TFIMO from consumers and local and international organizations (Bourgeault 1996, 74).

In total, eighty-six organizations, twenty-four of them women's groups, made submissions to the TFIMO. Only five of the submissions came from organizations representing racial minority groups, including the Union of Ontario Indians, the Multicultural Women's Centre, Women Working with Immigrant Women, and the Association of Iroquois and Allied Indians (TFIMO 1987, 273). Ironically, this was a period in Ontario of intense political organizing by women of colour and of the proliferation of community, provincial, and national groups devoted to gaining political rights for immigrant women of colour (Pierson and Chaudhuri 1993). Groups such as the National Organization of Immigrant and Visible Minority Women, the Congress of Black Women, the United Council of Filipino Associations of Canada, the Women's Committee of the Canadian Ethno-Cultural Council, the Chinese Canadian National Council, and Intercede, an advocacy organization for foreign domestic-workers all endeavoured in this period to provide services to marginalized women and to advocate for them on a number of fronts (Agnew 1996, 111). Struggles around racism in the feminist movement also moved to the fore. The National Action Committee on the Status of Women (NAC) had been pressured by women of colour to add an immigrant and visible minority women's committee, and organizers of Toronto's International Women's Day celebrations began, in the wake of intense criticism, to pursue a more antiracist organizational structure and politics. Feminists of colour identified racist dynamics as being endemic to many white-dominated feminist services and organizations (Findlay 1993, 208).

White-feminist activism was being increasingly directed toward gaining recognition and resources from the state. As Christina Gabriel (1996, 190) has noted, the province's responses to women of colour were "ad hoc" because this group could not be inserted neatly into either "race relations" or "women's policies" frameworks. Carmencita Hernandez (1988, 159), an activist who later served on a College of Midwives advisory board, observed, "There was no policy regarding visible minority women. As women we were not targeted by policies and programs of the OWD [Ontario Women's Directorate]; as visible minorities, we were lumped together with men by the Race Relations Directorate." A 1984 Royal Commission on Equality in Employment had identified four groups – women, visible minorities, Native people, and disabled persons – who had historically been disadvantaged and had suffered discrimination. Numerous policies and provincial bureaucracies like the Ontario Women's Directorate and the Race Relations Directorate ensued to address issues relating to the groups as defined by the commission. The defining concepts of these structures rendered them unable to deal with those whose identities overlapped these categories.

The legalization of midwifery was viewed as a "women's issue" and its successful implementation as a benefit to all women. Rarely does the *Report of the Task Force on the Implementation of Midwifery in Ontario* refer to social identities that complicate the category of "women." "Immigrant women," often an inferiorizing social category (Ng 1988), is invoked only in passing and only in terms of the "neediness" of such women. Even the advocacy group Women Working with Immigrant Women claimed in their submission to the TFIMO that "women from different cultures" needed midwifery care because they were averse to being treated by male physicians, thus reinscribing such women as subjects entrapped in gender-segregated patriarchal cultures (TFIMO 1987, 259). Moreover, the remedy promoted for this situation was care by women who were motivated by cross-race female empathy and who were, therefore, unimplicated in individual or systemic racism. Absent from the report, except in a statistical accounting of the province's nurses, is any reference to immigrant women of colour with midwifery training from their previous country of residence or to the barriers that might prevent them from benefiting from the province's attention to this "women's issue." White midwives and their supporters used their considerable skills and influence to produce an extraordinary number of submissions to the TFIMO. Women of colour, a group with a significant investment in the midwifery profession, were almost completely absent from the task force's report.

Accounting for Immigrant Midwives of Colour in the TFIMO Report
The *Report of the Task Force on the Implementation of Midwifery in Ontario* showed, inarguably, that immigrant midwives of colour were keenly interested in practising in the province. In a survey conducted in 1985 through the College of Nurses of Ontario, 4,514 registered nurses and registered nursing assistants reported that they had received midwifery training. It was estimated, however, that the actual number of nurses in the province with such training was between 6,000 and 7,200 (TFIMO 1987, 149). Approximately 35 percent of those who responded to the survey reported that they completed their midwifery education in the West Indies, India, or the Philippines. Among the total number of respondents with midwifery training, 621 desired to practise midwifery once legislation was in place. Only 110 of these had ever actually practised midwifery prior to coming to Canada. Of these

110, nearly 40 percent had practised in the "West Indies or the Philippines" (TFIMO 1987, 151). There are no data to indicate what portion of those respondents who said that they had previously practised in the United Kingdom or the "United Kingdom and another country," or who had indicated the category "other," were women of colour. However, among those immigrant midwives of colour interviewed for this study, seven out of seventeen or 41 percent had studied and/or practised midwifery in the United Kingdom. These data suggest that perhaps half or more of those who had been trained in midwifery, had practised before coming to Canada, and wished to resume practice were women of colour.

Estimates of the number of "racial-minority" women who were interested in practising the profession are complicated by post-1985 trends in immigration. Immigration to Canada from Europe accounted for 77 percent of immigrants in 1967. In 1987 only 22 percent of immigrants were Europeans. In 1987, immigration from South and Central America (including the Caribbean) quadrupled from 1967 rates (Task Force on Access to Professions and Trades in Ontario 1989, 12). Nearly 40 percent of Chinese immigrants, who comprise 26 percent of adults in "visible minority" groups, arrived in the years between 1982 and 1991. And similarly, nearly 40 percent of immigrants from the Philippines arrived in the years between 1982 and 1991, although they comprise only 7 percent of the total "visible minority" group (Statistics Canada 1999). In addition, in the period immediately preceding the legalization of midwifery, one-third of all Filipinas, as well as one-third of all black women, were working as health care professionals (Boyd 1992, 303), suggesting that immigrant women from the South may have been more likely to have training as health care workers, including midwifery training.[16]

The 110 women, probably half or more of whom were women of colour who had previously practised midwifery and who, in the College of Nurses survey, expressed an interest to do so again, must be considered carefully here. The data indicate significant confluences between nurses with midwifery training and those women engaged in re-emergent midwifery. According to the TFIMO report (TFIMO 1987, 343), these 110 nurses had, almost uniformly, performed the entire range of midwifery functions named in the survey. In addition, they had practised in a variety of settings and a notably high proportion – 71.3 percent – had conducted home births. The report also showed that, while this group envisioned midwifery as a nursing specialty with independent status, they were not wedded to the idea of nursing training as a prerequisite for hospital privileges for midwives in Ontario (TFIMO 1987, 382). Statistics for the cohort of all 621 of those who wished to practise (with and without experience) showed that nearly half supported the right of non-nurse-midwives to practise in the province both in and out of hospitals and that an overwhelming majority supported the right of all qualified midwives to conduct home births – positions not supported by their own provincial nursing organizations (TFIMO 1987, 382).

The data collected for the *Report of the Task Force on the Implementation of Midwifery in Ontario* offered the only knowledge available at the time about the skills and aspirations of immigrant midwives of colour. These statistics, as well as data about the philosophies and skills of foreign-trained midwives of colour, belie alarmist claims such as those made subsequently by the members of the Midwifery Task Force of Ontario who, it can be argued, entirely misread the TFIMO report. In a quote that resonates with racist discourses of immigrant invasion and usurpation, the civilized mission of midwifery is seen as being overrun by the uncivilized:

> It is important to remembers [sic] when we consider ongoing challenge testing that according to the 1987 survey in the Report of the Task Force on the Implementation of Midwifery in Ontario, there are approximately 4000 foreign-trained midwives working as nurses in Ontario. Of these approximately 600 would be interested in practising midwifery in Ontario. These are overwhelming numbers in comparison to the 50 or 60 practising midwives in Ontario today. There are concerns throughout Ontario that the soul of midwifery could be jeopardized by such a large influx of foreign-trained midwives with a different philosophy of continuity of care, choice of birthplace, and informed choice, who would shape or alter the approach of midwifery care simply as a result of their numbers.[17] (Matthews and Thatcher 1992, 21)

Even with the evidence of the TFIMO report proving the concept false, the project of integrating midwifery into the health care system became infused with the idea that foreign-trained midwives were philosophically opposed to the Ontario model of midwifery care. Midwifery activists and policy makers who supported them held firmly to the argument that foreign-trained midwives would endanger the project. Such an assertion also served to delineate the boundary between midwives' "turf" and that occupied by nurses. A member of the Interim Regulatory Council on Midwifery (IRCM), the first institutional precursor to the College of Midwives, commented:

> The issue of preserving the full model of care wasn't designed with any conscious intent to exclude anybody, as much as it was designed with conscious intent to protect ourselves against the College of Nurses, who initially wouldn't have wanted a home birth model ... The foreign-trained midwife thing for the IRCM ... wasn't a matter of "foreign," it wasn't a matter of "foreign" at all. It was people who didn't have the home birth experience. Because without the people having had that home birth experience

in the program, we couldn't protect home birth and that was really, really important to the model itself. (Interview no. 25)

Despite documentation demonstrating the wide scope of their former practice and indications of some degree of philosophical congruence between the Ontario midwifery movement and those nurses with midwifery training from abroad, the TFIMO report painted foreign-trained practitioners as effectively obsolete. It took pains to emphasize one aspect of what the College of Nurses of Ontario survey had reported: that the training of those who wished to practise after legislation had been obtained, for the most part, before 1970, and was therefore "outdated" (TFIMO 1987, 148). There was no recognition that, for those working as labour and delivery nurses, temporal distance from midwifery training and practice did not necessarily signal inferior midwifery skills. To claim so is to deny any confluence between obstetrical nursing knowledge and midwifery, a claim that cannot logically be substantiated. My research with immigrant midwives of colour who worked as labour and delivery nurses demonstrates that their midwifery qualifications distinguished them in the hospital setting as especially skilled, and even prompted doctors to allow them to manage deliveries alone in some institutions. However, in the end, the report concluded, "foreign-trained midwives" would probably need to repeat their basic midwifery education (TFIMO 1987, 346).

The designation of foreign-trained midwives' knowledge as obsolete had a negative impact on both white women and women of colour. For the latter, it replicated a racist legacy of the inferiorization of the credentials of nurses of colour in Canada (Calliste 1993) and became yet another roadblock in a system structured to limit their occupational mobility.

Few if any immigrant midwives of colour saw the necessity to make a special case with the task force for their integration into practice in the province. As my research shows, many were unaware of the impending legislation and those who were aware may have believed that their nursing organizations would protect their interests. Regrettably, they did not testify on their own behalf before the Task Force on the Implementation of Midwifery in Ontario, and their interests went unrepresented for the entire formative period of the midwifery profession in the province. But the TFIMO report did not formulate insuperable barriers for foreign-trained midwives. It recommended the initiation of a Midwifery Integration Program as "a means for the best qualified midwives, maternal/child nurses, and others to integrate into the regulated profession of midwifery" (TFIMO 1987, 153). It outlined a straightforward procedure in which anyone with twelve months of residency in Ontario as a citizen or permanent resident, English proficiency, and "educational preparation or significant experience in midwifery, maternal/infant nursing or medicine" (TFIMO 1987, 152) could undergo examinations leading to Ontario certification. The government-appointed bodies that were charged with the implementation of midwifery, and that were controlled largely by white midwifery practitioners, would reformulate these earlier policies in ways that worked to exclude women of colour. How this occurred and which purposes were served by exclusion will be explored in the next chapter.

2
Midwifery in Ontario:
A Counter-History

> The simple questions we should be asking are: who are places
> for, whom do they exclude, and how are these prohibitions
> maintained in practice?
>
> – David Sibley, *Geographies of Exclusion*

Dominant definitions of racism persist; perhaps the most widespread of these is the belief that racism is primarily an expression of personal prejudice. As Ruth Frankenberg (1993, 139) has reasoned, "Essentialist racism – particularly intentional, explicit racial discrimination – remains ... paradigmatic of racism." This dominant definition renders institutional and structural forms of racism difficult to discern. David Goldberg (1993, 98) argues that to understand the proliferation of racisms and the tenacity of racialized social formations, we need to articulate a definition of racisms as individual and institutional practices that "involve promoting exclusions, or the actual exclusions of people in virtue of their being deemed members of different racial groups, however racial groups are taken to be constituted." Departing fundamentally from the personal prejudice model of racism, Goldberg insists that intentionality cannot be the only grounds upon which individual or institutional practices can be judged to be racist. Rather, these practices must be judged on the basis of the effects they produce. Institutions, says Goldberg (99), can reasonably be presumed to be racist or to promote forms of racism when "institutional practice gives rise to racially patterned exclusionary or discriminatory outcomes, no matter the institutional aims, and the institution does little or nothing to avoid, diminish, or alleviate these outcomes." The grounds for exclusion are of utmost importance in this formulation, because they often appear as a "patterned by-product of bureaucratization" rationalized as the inevitable effect of the implementation of professional standards, prudent economic measures, or expedient politics

(98). Systemic practices of racist exclusion have largely supplanted ideological or biological discourses of racial inferiority and now constitute the most common forms of racism (Anthias and Yuval-Davis 1992; Essed 1991).

The cataloguing of exclusions in this chapter makes visible the spatial practices of the social movement to legalize midwifery in Ontario, as well as those of midwifery-related, state-funded regulatory bodies and midwifery's professional organization. Explicating Henri Lefebvre's concept, Edward Soja (1996, 66) describes spatial practice as "producing a spatiality that 'embraces production and reproduction, and the particular locations ... and spatial sets ... characteristic of each social formation.'" In other words, spaces of human sociality are not naturally occurring but require constant vigilance and a variety of repetitive moves to secure their reproduction, usually through practices of exclusion. In the case at hand, spatial practice can be understood to be about the production of spaces hospitable to white women and the exercise and consolidation of group power that may be named as "whiteness" (Lipsitz 1998; Frankenberg 1993).

The Interim Regulatory Council on Midwifery, Curriculum Design Committee, and Midwifery Integration Planning Project 1989-93

On 19 May 1989, thirteen members were appointed by provincial Order-in-Council to serve on an Interim Regulatory Council on Midwifery (IRCM) that would formulate policy leading to regulation (Ontario Interim Regulatory Council on Midwifery 1990, 1). The members included health care professionals and consumers. The IRCM was chaired by lawyer Mary Eberts, who had chaired the TFIMO. The *Report of the Task Force on the Implementation of Midwifery in Ontario* had indicated that midwives could not be appointed to any governing council until they were legally registered in the province, and it had recommended the appointment of a committee to "provide liaison and advice" to the Council. The liaison committee, stipulated to be constituted of "students in the Midwifery Integration Program and foreign-trained midwives waiting to present their credentials for recognition" (TFIMO 1987, 21), was selected and directed by the Association of Ontario Midwives and was composed of the organization's most politically involved members (Bourgeault 1996, 85). Remunerated on a per diem basis by the province, the liaison committee members functioned in a capacity almost identical to that of the Council's official members.[1] Foreign-trained midwives never received representation on the committee.

With one exception, the IRCM and the midwives' liaison committee were a white and privileged group (Ford 1992, 1). The awareness of this fact did not seem to prompt much introspection, nor did it diminish their sense of being on a pioneering mission. Council members found participation in the widely celebrated process a heady experience and one in which their own participation constituted a sort of heroism. One white Council member, a long-time midwifery activist, told me, "There was so much, um, sort of, you know 'The world is watching you' kind of thing that surrounded all those early days at the IRCM and the release of the [TFIMO] midwifery report, [which] all led to this kind of 'Oh, my God, can you believe it, we've actually done it.' And I think that a lot of us got very blinded by that attention and status that went with that" (Interview no. 27). However "blinded" Council members might have been, they were not entirely unaware of their own homogeneity. Such awareness, however, in no way blunted their desire to retain their seats on the Council and the attendant power to enact policy for the new profession. This member also recalled that "there was talking right from the beginning [...] that there was this awareness that it was not a representative group. That not only were we more or less, with the exception of Murray Enkin, in a certain age range, all white, all of a certain educational level ... I mean, it was appalling how homogeneous a group we were. So that got raised, but it was, ... there was never anybody really, uh, willing to take a strong stand [...] No one ever said, 'I'll come off the committee if you'll put a woman of colour in my place'" (Interview no. 27).

The only Council member who did not fit the profile described above was Jesse Russell. Russell, a Métis woman from Thunder Bay, had worked as a policy analyst on Aboriginal women's issues, providing services to the Ontario Women's Directorate (Ontario Interim Regulatory Council on Midwifery 1991a, 3). One interviewee described Russell as "the only voice that brought a different community perspective around the table" (Interview no. 27). "Russell," claimed the same Council member, "never felt like she belonged." Russell's only committee appointment on the Council was to the equity committee, a body not mandated by the final HPLR report but that had been formed at her urging (Ontario IRCM 1993a, 10). Russell's participation on the Council was focused unwaveringly on the impact on Aboriginal women of the impending regulation of midwifery, and she exercised considerable influence, as I will show, in bringing to the table the contentious and uncomfortable issue of jurisdiction over Aboriginal midwifery. One Council member indicated that it was the political pressure of Aboriginal groups that forced the Council to acquiesce, ultimately, to the exemption of Aboriginal midwives from the legislation.

The Curriculum Design Committee on the Development of Midwifery Education in Ontario (CDC) and the Midwifery Integration Planning Project (MIPP), two groups that functioned separately from but concurrently with the IRCM, enacted policies that took significant exclusionary turns. The CDC, formed in 1989, was empowered by the provincial government to develop a midwifery curriculum and to propose options for a site for a midwifery education program. In addition, the CDC was to recommend a program for the integration of those with prior midwifery experience. While the CDC's decisions would have a significant impact on foreign-trained midwives who expressed an interest in practising, the impact was more profoundly felt by women of colour. No immigrant women of colour, however, were appointed to the committee and no organizations representing the interests of these women offered submissions.[2] Like the TFIMO, the CDC referenced only midwifery data from Europe. However, it diverged from the TFIMO in reformulating its recommendations regarding foreign-trained midwives so as to effectively exclude them from participation in an integration program intended to incorporate those with midwifery expertise into the newly legalized profession.

The CDC retained the TFIMO policy of baccalaureate preparation as the educational standard for midwifery practice but abandoned its recommendation that a twelve- to eighteen-month diploma stream be available for nurses with university-level training. This decision had exclusionary consequences for foreign-trained midwives across the board. Baccalaureate preparation for nurses and midwives is exceedingly rare worldwide. "Visible minority" immigrant women are more likely to be university trained than those born in Canada (15 percent versus 10 percent) (Statistics Canada 1995, 58). This statistic may not, however, represent the educational attainments of nurses in this group, many of whom received their training in countries where, as in Canada, baccalaureate preparation for nursing has, until only recently, not been the norm. In the period under discussion, approximately 14 percent of Canadian nurses held baccalaureate nursing degrees (Sedivy-Glasgow 1992, 28). However, some statistics indicate that less than one-half of 1 percent of all foreign-trained nurses with formal midwifery education were university educated (TFIMO 1987, 331). Having been eliminated from the program designed to integrate practising midwives into the health care system, most foreign-trained midwives would have to augment or repeat their prior education to gain entrance to practice.[3] The discriminatory nature of the baccalaureate requirement can be viewed as particularly grievous given the fact that the CDC and the MIPP did not require applicants to the Michener Institute Pre-registration Program, which integrated currently practising midwives into the health care system, to have or complete a baccalaureate credential (Schatz 1992).

The TFIMO (1987, 153) had designated that the integration process be open to "the best qualified midwives, maternal/child nurses, and others." It recommended that "an integration program be developed as quickly as possible to meet the needs of those midwifery practitioners with current experience in Ontario" (Curriculum Design Committee 1990, 12). A second CDC (1990, 38) recommendation had a more direct exclusionary impact on immigrant midwives. Members of this group, identified as "midwives without Ontario experience" in the TFIMO report rather than as "foreign-trained midwives," were to apply to the future College of Midwives to have their credentials assessed.[4] Five years would pass before this was a possibility.

Appointed in October 1990, the Midwifery Integration Planning Project took up where the CDC had left off. Identical to its predecessor in its racial homogeneity, the MIPP's mandate was to formulate the procedure by which practising midwives would be assessed and licensed. In their third meeting, MIPP members recommended that to be eligible for the integration project, candidates must have practised two years out of the previous six in Ontario (Midwifery Integration Planning Project 1990, 2). The requirement succeeded in keeping out and raising the ire of some apprentice, newly practising, and rural midwives. The greatest impact was felt by the immigrant midwives of colour; they were the least likely to have had Ontario experience and therefore, despite other qualifications, the least likely to qualify for the planned integration program and for immediate access to practice. The Ontario practice requirement firmly inscribed a normative national/racial identity onto professional midwifery and delayed for years the entry of women of colour into the profession.

Midwives of colour were less likely to be located within the social geography of the nearly monoracial Ontario midwifery community. As a consequence, they were also less likely to establish apprenticeships that could link them to the social networks where midwifery was in demand and where clients were able to pay the fees necessary to sustain a midwife in full-time practice. Some midwives of colour did, however, deliver babies within immigrant communities, but their clients' low incomes kept their practices small. One white midwife related in an interview how she had, in the early 1990s, struck a partnership with a midwife who had emigrated from a Latin American country. The fees the women were paid by their working-class Latin American immigrant clientele were often well below the going rate of six hundred dollars and therefore both continued to work part time – a situation that prevented them from accumulating the number of births necessary to be considered for the Michener Institute program.

As Sherene Razack (1999) has argued, immigrant people of colour in white settler societies are always construed as a threat to the racial order. Even when legally allowed to dwell within such societies, they are subject to surveillance and their "goodness" is the counterpoint invoked to highlight the "badness" of undocumented immigrants. Under these circumstances, it is not surprising that immigrant people of colour become hyper-vigilant about not breaking the law. Immigrant midwives of colour are no exception. Prior to legalization, these women feared legal prosecution and deportation if they practised in the legal limbo characterizing the period (Burtch 1994). Stories of deportation of immigrants of colour and their construction as criminals are daily fare in the Canadian press.[5] And even documented immigrants, argues Sherene Razack (1999, 171), speaking of her own experience, "can still be confused with the unruly mob and suspected of treason at worst, of failing to conform to respectable codes of behaviour at best."

Midwives of colour related in interviews that they strictly avoided using their clinical skills even when they were requested to attend out-of-hospital births of friends and relatives. As one Indo-Caribbean midwife put it, "You're coming from Third World countries, from war-torn countries, whatever, or you're just coming because you think the grass is greener here. Can you imagine coming to this country and working as a midwife illegally? We so want to do things the right way. I don't think they [midwifery officials] envision what it means to come here as an immigrant [and] do something illegally" (Interview no. 8). An Afro-Caribbean midwife told me, "I didn't want to jeopardize my status to become a midwife because I wanted to be a Canadian" (Interview no. 6).

IRCM Members' Explanatory Schema of Exclusion

Two out of the three Interim Regulatory Council on Midwifery (IRCM) members interviewed for this study admitted that the midwifery integration process had been a racially exclusionary one. They all used similar explanatory strategies to rationalize the exclusions, but only one interviewee demonstrated significant remorse. Three discursive devices enabled these IRCM members and many others to rationalize and ultimately acquiesce to the racist exclusion that they observed. These were the "heroic tale" of midwifery, "white solidarity," and "inoculation."

The first, and most indispensable of these, is the interviewees' participation in what has already been identified as the "heroic tale" of the re-emergence of midwifery. Central to the heroic narrative offered by midwifery activists was the claim that exclusionary strategies that led to the legalization of midwifery were justified both because of the anticipated benefits to women and because midwifery's (largely medical) adversaries were extraordinarily powerful (Davidson 1997). Recounting her own moral struggles with the exclusions that she observed, one IRCM member told me:

> The more I met women who it affected, the more I realized that there was something wrong with it and the more disillusioned I became. It was a constant struggle in my mind and not just me, there were other community members on the IRCM who felt very similar to me. There was a constant feeling of "You know why you've done it this way" ... and this will go down in history as being an absolutely remarkable coup for the women's health movement and the childbirth movement in this country ... But there are pieces of that that probably should have been re-examined along the way. Now the argument for why they weren't re-examined ... was always that there were these other forces that were powerful, that were gonna get us if we weren't careful, if we didn't show solidarity and unity amongst ourselves that we wouldn't ... it was always held before us like a carrot. (Interview no. 27)

Using what I call the "forces of evil" excuse – an unmistakable "race to innocence" (Fellows and Razack 1998) strategy in which the claim to oppressed status is used to deflect knowledge of one's own dominant positioning – another IRCM member rationalized exclusionary practice in the following way: "I mean it happened that there weren't people with different skin colours doing this. And the problem was protection of the model and vulnerability of the model. You have no idea what kind of beating we took from the medical profession in those years and how vulnerable we were to getting absolutely killed ... If we weren't careful in registering, in the preregistration process we exposed the professions to inadequacies of practice that left us vulnerable to vultures just waiting to kill or waiting to pick up the spoils ..." (Interview no. 25).

If the "heroic tale" constituted the theory that rationalized exclusion in the pre-integration period, then "white solidarity" was the practice through which exclusion materialized. Although the appointments to the IRCM had been made by Health Minister Elinor Caplan, many of the recommendations had come from midwives and midwifery activists (Bourgeault 1996, 83). Some women who had been appointed had themselves been midwifery consumers, and they were zealously loyal to the midwives who attended their births. As well, the liaison committee members were all prominent midwives. Solidarity in this case had a number of complex dimensions. IRCM members whom I interviewed indicated that they were reluctant to abandon allegiance to those with whom they shared both the politics of and the significant personal event of childbirth. Said one Council member, "We were supporters, they knew we loved them and that we'd back them. Some of them had delivered our babies" (Interview no. 27).

In the IRCM and elsewhere, intense interpersonal links, formed under conditions of ideological commonality and struggle among women whose class backgrounds and racial identities were extraordinarily congruent, rendered any critique of white racial privilege unthinkable, if not traitorous, to the midwifery cause. The solidarity expressed here is a form of what Christine Sleeter (1996, 261) calls "white racial bonding" – a set of "interactions that have the purpose of affirming a common stance on race-related issues, legitimating particular interpretations of oppressed groups, and drawing we-they boundaries." Such interactions, Sleeter (263) posits, invite white people to signal their solidarity with the dominant racial group. To refuse to participate in these rituals, she argues, is to risk losing the approval and friendship of one's peers. Breaking the ranks of white sisterhood also posed the risk of losing one's self. In psychoanalytic terms, argues Carol Schick (1998, 115), "The desire is to see oneself ... as good ... with the fantasies covering over or forgetting parts of the narrative that do not coincide." Coming to grips with exclusion would have meant an end to these women's sense of themselves as benevolent and unimplicated in relations of domination –

notions fundamental to their participation in midwifery-related work. Finally, while it may be difficult to envision this "solidarity" as a de facto consolidation of white privilege and not merely as loyalty to a cause, precisely this kind of envisioning is needed if white women are to cease reproducing relations of domination.

Managing Difference: The IRCM Equity Committee

A third device used by Interim Regulatory Council on Midwifery members to rationalize exclusion, and one that effectively "inoculated" the midwifery project against charges of discriminatory practice, was the foregrounding of the accomplishments of the IRCM's equity committee. In a provocative essay, Chéla Sandoval (1997, 88) outlines several figures of French social and literary critic Roland Barthes's "rhetoric of supremacy" which "shape and inhabit not only the most obedient and deserving citizen/subject, but also even the most rebellious agent of social change." The first of Barthes's figures is "the inoculation." In this process, "modest doses of dissimilarity" are introduced, providing the subject's consciousness with a cautious exposure to forms of difference that can be "taken in, tamed and domesticated" (Sandoval 1997, 89). Having ingested the serum of difference, the subject becomes "immune" to difference's more virulent strains and to their threat to the very tissue of subjecthood – itself contingent on the difference it seeks to deflect. This process is very evident in official midwifery publications and in other materials written by midwifery supporters that touted the establishment of an equity committee as evidence of Ontario midwifery's commitment to anti-oppression politics. This commitment was characterized by midwifery officials and supporters as without parallel among regulated health professionals in the province (Ford 1991, 1993; Ontario IRCM 1991b, 1992a, 1992b, 1993; Shroff 1997). Before returning to this point, I will summarize the work of the equity committee.

In January 1990 the IRCM was presented with a mandate for an equity committee that was to "ensure that the proposed College of Midwives is responsive to different groups who are interested in midwifery as a profession or as a service ... focusing on varied language and cultural groups, disadvantaged women and women in institutions" (Ontario IRCM 1990a, 4). The committee, which had been proposed by Jesse Russell and which included her as well as three other IRCM members, was not mandated by the provincial government and was something of an aberration among other professions that had undergone the Health Professions Legislation Review process.

Between 1990 and 1993, the committee conducted a series of consultations across the province intended to elicit input from marginalized groups about access to midwifery care and practice. The groups included Aboriginal women, women with disabilities, immigrant and refugee women, and Mennonite, teen, and lesbian women. However, the committee focused the bulk of its attention on the concerns expressed by various First Nations communities. At least half the pages of the committee's published "equity reports" were devoted to consultations done in Northern and Northwestern Ontario, the Akwesasne First Nations Reserve in Eastern Ontario, and the Six Nations Reserve near Brantford. It is entirely logical that the committee's focus should have been directed at Aboriginal women's childbearing, given Jesse Russell's intense passion on the issue and her position as initiator of the committee (Ontario IRCM 1992e, 2). Russell's initiatives, along with political organizing among Aboriginal people, brought pressure upon both the IRCM and the Ministry of Health to exempt Aboriginal midwives from regulation under the pending Regulated Health Professions Act.

First Nations Midwifery and Ontario Midwives: Tracking Exemption and Redemption

By September 1990, the Ontario Native Women's Association had adopted a resolution at its annual assembly calling for "steps to insure that the needs and concerns of Aboriginal women are brought to the attention of the provincial government regarding midwifery" (Ontario IRCM 1991a, 3). In a letter dated 7 May 1991 to then Health Minister Frances Lankin, James Morris, deputy grand chief of the Nishnawbe-Aski Nation, stated: "It is important that regulations and legislation do not obstruct existing traditional midwifery practices within the Native communities and their desires to revitalize any midwifery practices in the future." Lankin received another letter soon after from Equay-wuk, the Native group representing Nishnawbe women from the twenty-eight communities within Northwestern Ontario (Terry and Calm Wind 1994), expressing concern that the legislation would not benefit Aboriginal women in the North (Melvin, 10 May 1991). However, the strongest statement on the impact of midwifery legislation on Aboriginal communities came in August 1991 from the Ontario Native Women's Association:

> It is obviously evident the social issues and conditions in Native Communities ... are the result of Natives not being in the control of their affairs ... Again it seems that the same mistakes are reoccurring with the midwifery issue. In the report that was prepared by the task force [TFIMO], it is clear that once again, government agencies are assuming control of issues that clearly affect Native people and Native communities. The task force has only suggested that Native people ... will receive special treatments such as flexible admission policies. This clearly is not enough. Native people ultimately have to be in control [of] their own affairs to improve the social

issues ... It would be counterproductive to continue with any strategies which involve Natives and Native communities without the involvement of Native people. (Ontario Native Women's Association 1991, 8)

Equay-wuk and the Nishnawbe-Aski Nation also submitted a brief to the Ontario Ministry of Health with recommendations for the protection of Aboriginal midwives and against any obstruction of their practices by legislation, regulation, or education policies related to Ontario midwifery (Equay-wuk Women's Group and Nishnawbe-Aski Nation 1991, 8). The overwhelming impulse among Native organizations was to gain exemption for Aboriginal midwives and traditional Native healers from the pending Regulated Health Professions Act. Given the anticipated impact of the RHPA, exemption was the very condition upon which Aboriginal midwifery and other forms of traditional healing might be protected and expanded (Couchie and Nabigon 1997). On 30 October 1991, representatives from the Ministry of Health met with Native groups, and an agreement was reached that would exempt Aboriginal midwives and healers from the Act. Members of the IRCM were not invited to attend the meeting. Following both the enactment of an exemption clause and vigorous statements from Native communities asserting Aboriginal control over midwifery, the equity committee continued to visit and collect information in at least five other Native communities.[6]

Despite the time, resources, and attention devoted to Aboriginal issues through these consultations, their impact on Aboriginal women's access to midwifery practice through the mechanisms created by the legislative process was minimal. In July of 1993, less than six months before final proclamation of the Midwifery Act, the Ontario Native Women's Association declared that

the current university programme offering a Bachelor of Midwifery degree lacks a cultural component in its curriculum design specific to Aboriginal needs. It is our belief that ineffective and inefficient consultation with Aboriginal communities and organizations has been made in the early stages of curriculum design to allow for a cultural component.

A report on the admission process [to the Preregistration Program] ... has indicated that out of a total of 149 applicants, 2 were Aboriginal women. Of the 80 successful candidates, one was Aboriginal. The accepted Aboriginal candidate does not reside in the province of Ontario. The reasons for this inequity remain questionable, however, there may be some connection to the fact that the admissions committee was comprised largely of foreign midwives unfamiliar with Canadian history and the position of Aboriginal peoples.

In any effect, the inequity generated within the Michener Institute program has been interpreted as grossly inadequate, given that Aboriginal peoples have the highest birth rates per capita in comparison to Caucasian women or women of other ethnic minority groups. (Thomas 1993, 27)

These issues were flagged as far back as 1991. At an equity committee consultation with Native residents of Sioux Lookout conducted that year, participants asked the committee to curtail their presentation on the IRCM so that they might present their own issues. One of the speakers told the Committee, "Natives are always put in the position of having to respond to and deal with legislation that already exists." Those present called for two seats on midwifery bodies for Native women in Northern Ontario and a subcommittee of Native people to address Native concerns. They also suggested that Native women should be conducting consultations about the way midwifery would be implemented in northern communities (Ontario IRCM 1991c, 10). Native people used the consultations as a forum to express opinions on a variety of reproductive health issues and to send a strong message of displeasure to the provincial government about a legislative process that seemed to circumvent other policies relating to Aboriginal self-government. For the Native communities involved in the consultations, the equity committee provided a fortuitous opportunity to amplify a burgeoning political protest.

Canada's attempts to westernize the childbirth practices of First Nations peoples are a paradigm of the cultural violence enacted through the imposition of Western birthing practices on Native populations (O'Neil and Kaufert 1990, 1995; Thomas 1993). Such colonial interventions produced a loss of local knowledge and autonomy and disrupted complex social links. This issue is of vital concern, and I do not in any way mean, through this critique, to diminish its importance. However, inasmuch as the IRCM, the MIPP, and the CDC do not appear to have enacted policies that fostered Native women's participation in midwifery, and inasmuch as Native organizations seemed to want to disentangle their communities entirely from the imposed web of midwifery legislation, how are we to understand the equity committee's devoting the majority of its scarce resources to Aboriginal issues even after the Aboriginal exemption clause had been achieved?

There are a number of ways to answer this query. To begin with, as Carol Schick (1998, 243) has observed in another context, it is safer for white groups making claims to multicultural sensitivity to promote the equality of those who offer no imminent threat to their dominance than to champion those whose threat is more immediate. In distinct contrast to numerically significant, urban-dwelling immigrant midwives of colour, the few Aboriginal midwives practising in geographical locations outside the major Ontario cities where midwifery activity was centred hardly threatened to overtake the midwifery movement. They often pursued parallel, rather than competing, routes to midwifery practice, routes that constituted only a minimal threat to the Ontario midwifery project. Aboriginal people were also seen to be docile political partners. In the past political experience of some IRCM members, one interviewee explained, coalition with Aboriginal people was "not ... as volatile as some of the alliances that have been made with groups around race" (Interview no. 27). In contrast to other feminist cross-race initiatives, the equity committee's motives and benevolence seemed unlikely to be challenged by Native groups defending Aboriginal midwifery.

The concern with Aboriginal issues can be viewed as a benevolent venture, but as Barbara Heron (1999, 88) argues, the performance of benevolent acts for the racialized other is never simply good or bad but represents a "complex mixture of relations and effects." Such acts confer a moral status on those who perform them. As Heron states, the performance of these acts is key to the construction of the white female bourgeois figure who constantly requires "moral superiority, a self-image as a saviour and self-satisfaction through favourable (to us) comparison with Others." Midwifery's championing of Aboriginal concerns could only be construed as a moral and antiracist venture through a disavowal of the uneven relations of power between white midwives and Native communities. This was accomplished in two ways: first, through the idealization of Aboriginal people, a strategy which purports to invert oppressive constructs but which succeeds only in reproducing the binary categories of "Indian" and "white" within the Canadian nation (Légère 1995, 356); and second, through the promulgation of a set of "redemption discourses" in which white midwifery activists imagined themselves (and not Aboriginal people) as the saviours of Aboriginal midwifery. The ameliorative effects of Ontario midwifery's concern with Aboriginal peoples are minor when compared with what such a concern yielded in terms of producing politically efficacious subjectivities for midwives and those involved in midwifery implementation.

Any unravelling of the complex relationship between Aboriginal peoples and Ontario midwifery as it was represented by the Interim Regulatory Council on Midwifery must begin with Jesse Russell, a Métis woman and the only racialized minority person to serve on that body. Russell's dual positioning as both idealized "other" and feminist activist rendered her claims of inequity and exclusion difficult for Council members to dismiss. She was the very embodiment of a subaltern group whose idealization had been an important discursive strategy in the re-emergence of midwifery in North America. If, as some activists argued, midwives across time and space were the heroines of a drama in which "female healers champion the natural, resist technology and are instinctively in sympathy with the childbearing woman" (Treichler 1990, 118), then participation in the enactment of midwifery legislation that stood to endanger indigenous Canadian childbearing practices threatened to unsettle the ontological ground upon which the midwifery movement's identity had been built.

The North American childbirth reform movement has long idealized indigenous birth practitioners, imagining them to possess uncorrupted knowledge of the female body (Nestel 1995). This idealization typifies the process of "eating the Other" described by bell hooks (1992, 25), in which "a contemporary longing for the 'primitive' is expressed by projection onto the Other of a sense of plenty, bounty, a field of dreams."[7] That this process was at work here is confirmed by the equity committee member who relates, in this passage, what can only be described as a perfect paradigm of not only eating a particularly delectable "other" but disgorging her as well for voyeuristic display:

> I mean there was a kind of momentum that got started early on, and the momentum was around this incredible, extremely selfish on our parts, but this incredible cultural phenomenon, which is how birth is handled in Aboriginal communities, or was handled, that some of us were just learning about for the first time. And we were awestruck and we were amazed and we were disgusted – one, that it was being lost and, two, you know our ancestors had contributed to its loss – all of those things, and that's where the guilt comes in. And I think that we were, we kind of rolled with that momentum, and we were having the opportunity to visit these, to have these incredible experiences. So that's when I say it was selfish. We were having these incredible cultural opportunities that every Canadian should have the experience of, and we rolled with it. We talked about it, we made briefs to the Aboriginal Commission on it. We brought people back with us and had smudge ceremonies at our meeting; it was a really a big kind of "happening." There wasn't anything equivalent from any of the other communities we talked to. (Interview no. 27)

In this speech, the responsibility of white settlers for the destruction of Aboriginal peoples gets a brief acknowledgment but the genocidal past is seemingly redressed and attendant guilt assuaged through the interviewee's reverential consumption of Aboriginality, a move that anthropologist Renato Rosaldo (1989, 108) has dubbed "imperialist nostalgia." Left unexamined are the contemporary relations of domination that construct the very encounter in which equity committee members were engaged.

Cultural theorist Philip J. Deloria (1998, 161) argues that countercultural movements of the late twentieth century have had a particular affinity for "Indianness," seeing identification with Aboriginal peoples as a way of moving their white identities "away from Americanness altogether to leap outside national boundaries, gesture at repudiating the nation, and offer what seemed a clear-eyed political critique."[8] The gesture seen here is one of repudiation of white IRCM members' implication in a racialized order in a belief that it could be willed away through practices of identification. However, as Leslie Roman (1997, 273) argues, such practices are linked to a set of "redemption discourses" that may have certain limited counter-hegemonic effects but which serve to reinscribe the identities of both dominant and subordinate subjects.

Some IRCM members believed that it was the equity committee that rescued traditional Aboriginal midwifery from threatened suppression under the pending Midwifery Act. In their presentation to the Royal Commission on Aboriginal Peoples in November of 1992, committee members Anne Rochon Ford and Vicki Van Wagner proclaimed that as "a result of the information we have brought back from communities we have visited, the Ontario government has noted the importance of a more equitable approach to any health professions legislative changes which will have an impact on Aboriginal people" (Ontario IRCM 1992g, 4). An IRCM member whom I interviewed reiterated this position succinctly in our interview. In response to my prodding about whether she thought the equity committee's emphasis on Aboriginal issues was justified, the member responded, "I mean, if we did nothing else successful we did the Aboriginal stuff. That came out of the equity committee. We literally turned that legislation on its head literally three days before it went in for third reading. They stopped the whole process and revised the legislation around Aboriginal issues because we had done that. That's one of the constructive things toward equity that we achieved" (Interview no. 25).

The midwifery movement's foregrounding of Aboriginal issues achieved two related, but slightly different, effects. The first of these was the creation of the inoculatory device described above. If midwifery activists can be seen as having rescued Aboriginal midwifery from extinction, then there exists exculpatory evidence against possible charges of racist exclusion of non-Aboriginal "others." But this strategy was useful not just in deflecting criticism from the outside; it also helped liberal-thinking IRCM members to resolve the contradiction that indelibly marked the re-emergence of midwifery: that the disqualification of racialized minority midwives helped secure the access of a small number of white women to the lucrative, newly legalized profession. It might be argued that Aboriginal midwifery was the site for a symbolic resolution of this troubling contradiction. This process is quite evident in the following quote, where an IRCM member's discursive strategy of simultaneously acknowledging exclusion and recuperating innocence is deployed: "We didn't learn enough and we didn't do it well enough and I agree with you in that respect. But *then*, we were just absolutely boggling every bloody mind in the health professions world at the time with how unbelievably progressive and audacious we were" (Interview no. 25).

"Immigrant and Refugee Women" in the Equity Reports

White midwives had been inferiorized by other health professionals and had been practising in a quasi-legal manner in the province. To counter this, they had long employed sophisticated discursive repertoires to promote the midwifery movement in the press and other public forums. Pending legislation had given them direct access to what Teun van Dijk (1993b, 45) calls "the means of production of public opinion." The widely circulated and referenced "equity reports" were foundational to securing midwifery's respectability. One discursive strategy employed by midwifery activists was to construct themselves as the saviours of Aboriginal people. And while far less attention was paid in the equity reports to "immigrant and refugee women" than to Native peoples, the scant eleven pages devoted to this over-determined group are no less instructive in demonstrating how this form of white representation works. As Richard Dyer (1997, 12) has argued, it is not just the deployment of stereotypes that achieves racial differentiation; this effect is achieved as well through "narrative structural positions, rhetorical tropes and habits of perception." In the case of the equity committee's *Midwifery and Immigrant and Refugee Women* report (Ontario IRCM 1993b), the narrative structure positions "immigrant and refugee women" as needy and white midwives who practise "culturally sensitive midwifery" as those capable of remedying their need. The report, through its very title, draws on a recognizable rhetorical trope that has come to signify "women of colour, women from Third World countries, women who do not speak English well and women who occupy lower positions in the occupational hierarchy" (Ng and Estable 1987, 29). The report reinscribed this trope and the racialization process by focusing on issues of victimization, including linguistic and cultural barriers to adequate obstetrical care, the negative obstetrical experiences of women who had undergone "female circumcision,"[9] and the difficulties faced by political refugees in dealing with authority figures.

By the admission of one equity committee member, participation by women of colour in the consultations upon which the report is based was scant. Unlike their consultations with Aboriginal people, for which the equity committee travelled to reserves and Native community agencies, the committee's meetings with women of colour required that these women come to them, a strategy that appears to have been less than efficacious. As one committee member put it, "Turnouts were almost always poor. There was poor reception on the other end of the line in a lot of cases and we didn't have the 'ins' that we needed. We weren't getting in and we weren't being welcomed" (Interview no. 27). This member admitted that committee members did not aggressively solicit input from women of colour and some of this avoidance was due to their wish to avoid "women's politics *à la* Toronto ... 1980s" (Interview no. 27), that is, the vigorous challenge that had been mounted by women of colour to the racism of feminist organizations in the city.

The reports were based, to some degree, on consultations that were individual and informal, and not specifically tied to the committee's activities. Some of what went into making the equity reports, specifically around immigrant women, "was sort of mixed up or tied in with personal consultations we had with individuals or with two or three women who [another Committee member] might have gone out with or I went out with or discussed, you know, in a break in a conference, all of that kind of stuff would have fed the things that are in there" (Interview no. 27). However, the majority of those who ended up consulting with the equity committee were midwives of colour, and contrary to what is represented in the reports, it appears that it was not victimization that they wanted to discuss: "Who actually ended up coming to most of the gatherings were foreign-trained midwives ... and all they wanted to talk about was access to training. And they had, you know, every reason in the world to be there and every reason in the world to be angry. You know, here they had an opportunity to get some of the people who were involved in making the legislation and get our ear, and we were caught because it wasn't what we were supposed to be doing" (Interview no. 27).

As Jane Flax (1993, 40) has noted, power produces "the appearance of a neutral resolution" by eliding truth claims that threaten to fragment a given discourse. Marginalization and silencing are some of the discursive practices that make such elisions possible. These women came to the equity committee with a truth claim that challenged the dominant epistemology in which women of colour were understood to be the needy recipients of midwifery care, and not its potential providers. What they lacked was the power to circulate such a challenge. The report specifies that the committee met with women who had "practised as midwives in their countries of origin and were anxious to practise here." This issue, claimed the report, was not in the mandate of the equity committee but was "in the jurisdiction of the Registration Committee" (Ontario IRCM 1993b, 2). Equity was in no way achieved through this route.[10]

In suppressing the access-to-practice issues raised by immigrant midwives of colour, the report enacts significant epistemic violence. Not only are the voices of immigrant midwives of colour introduced and then suppressed in the report through a bureaucratic sleight of hand, this elision is rendered normal through a reliance on racist discourses. Denied any competing formulation about their identities and in the absence of any listener positioned to receive their insurgent messages, "immigrant and refugee women" are effectively muted (Spivak 1988). They remain discursively constructed as a powerless and needy population while Ontario midwives are produced as those white middle-class female subjects capable of saving them. Within this economy of meaning, immigrant women of colour who are autonomous, competent, and sophisticated practitioners of midwifery are not just silenced, they are rendered unimaginable – virtual non-subjects. This was a construct of some value for those struggling to integrate midwifery into the health care system. Popular perceptions of midwifery as a primitive and discredited form of feminized care threatened the midwifery movement's struggle to foreground a new and respectable "professional midwife," configured as modern, university-educated, feminist, and therefore, in all likelihood, white. The presence in the province of thousands of trained midwives from Third World countries jeopardized that construction and made the confirmation of respectable subjectivities a matter of some urgency for those who supported the professionalization project.

The IRCM's equity committee was a contradictory project: the intentions of those who participated in it were to disrupt various forms of privilege and its actual effects guaranteed that privilege remained intact. Claiming to pursue equitable treatment within the re-emergence of midwifery, the equity committee reports reinscribed marginalized identities and secured dominant ones for white midwives. The pursuit of equity was not a power-sharing endeavour but rather constituted a project that very publicly produced white midwives as benevolent and rendered them apparently innocent of racist exclusions.

The Transitional Council of the College of Midwives of Ontario, 1993

The Transitional Council of the College of Midwives of Ontario (TCCMO) was created by Order-in-Council in February 1993 and was the immediate predecessor of the College of Midwives, which would become, with the passage of the Regulated Health Professions Act, the regulatory body of the midwifery profession in Ontario (Bourgeault 1996, 87). The TCCMO is of interest here because its composition reflected far more social diversity than had any midwifery organization or government-appointed body that preceded it. Unlike its Liberal predecessor, the newly elected New Democratic Party government embraced an aggressive equity agenda and proposed appointments to the Transitional Council that reflected representation of very specific constituencies. The five professional members were to include one Aboriginal midwife and one who was "foreign credentialed"[11] and the seven public members would comprise, in addition to three IRCM members who were to provide continuity, one Aboriginal member, one disabled woman, one consumer from Northern Ontario, and one "visible minority" member (Ontario IRCM 1992c, 3). The government exerted its authority in making the appointments. It acceded to the IRCM's recommendations vis-à-vis Aboriginal appointees; at the same time, it chose to appoint two women of colour – one professional member and one public member – neither of whom had previously been involved with the Ontario midwifery movement.

The composition of the Transitional Council reflected a more equitable representation of the province's "visible minority" population. This seemingly improved configuration had only a minor impact on the achievement of equity within the new profession for at least two important reasons. First, critical decisions had already been made about access of all foreign-trained midwives to the first cadre of practitioners. These guaranteed that immigrant midwives, among them substantial numbers of women of colour, would have a long and complicated route to practice. The presence of racialized minority women on the Transitional Council did not undo these important policy decisions. Second, unlike the IRCM, which had the arguably exciting task of imagining a new profession into being, the Transitional Council had the far more tedious task of writing the College's regulations and policies. Those Transitional Council members who had had no prior experience on midwifery bodies found themselves at a disadvantage in relation to this work; the majority of these new members without such experience were "visible minority" or Aboriginal appointments. One IRCM member interpreted the situation thus: "Because we were now dealing with technicalities and regulation and things of that nature, new consumer members, and I remember hearing this from people within a few months of its operation, were left in the dust. I mean as wonderful as their diversity and their contribution was, they didn't have a hope in hell of competing with the technical knowledge and in the technical tasks that were demanded of the Transitional Council" (Interview no. 25). As well as the disadvantage conferred upon them by lack of exposure to the midwifery politics that preceded the appointments, racialized minority women who served on midwifery-related councils and boards between 1993 and 1995 experienced significant marginalization and numerous forms of overt and covert racism.

Prior Learning Assessment and Access to Midwifery Practice for Immigrant Midwives of Colour

> Enchanted by the tantalizing image of Canada, professionals in various countries eagerly give up their jobs to immigrate to Canada. Often, they are granted residence visas based on a point-scoring system that recognizes academic qualifications and professional standing, as well as financial and social status. Consequently, these professionals immigrate believing that jobs abound in their various fields and that their professional expertise will be optimized

and appreciated. Once in Canada, their rosy expectations quickly prove to be illusions: they face tedious and expensive processes of credentials assessment and licensing, as well as barriers to employment. All too soon, the initial optimism and enthusiasm give way to disillusionment.

– Margaret Azuh, *Foreign-Trained Professionals*

The Task Force on Access to Professions and Trades in Ontario (TFAPTO) publicly identified exclusionary practices in the licensing procedures of professions in the province. In the report, entitled *Access!*, the task force cited long delays in gaining access to language and training programs, lack of financial support during retraining, and difficulties in qualifying for language programs as some of the barriers to professional practice (TFAPTO 1989, xv). It concluded that while all immigrants were affected by systemic barriers that were "administrative, economic and cultural in origin," "minority and ethnic groups" suffered disproportionately (TFAPTO 1989,4).

Despite the bold and thorough recommendations of the *Access!* report and the subsequent establishment by the then Ministry of Citizenship of an Access to Professions and Trades Unit, barriers to professional practice continue to be a contentious public issue in Ontario. In 1999, a series in the *Toronto Star* focused attention on the fight of immigrant professionals to obtain professional credentials, citing uneven assessment practices, high costs, and the dissemination of misleading employment information to potential immigrants as among the barriers to accreditation (Hurst 1999; Murray 1999a, 1999b, 1999c). Indeed, the issue of credential recognition for internationally trained professionals has been the focus of government bodies and advocacy groups in Ontario in recent years. A regional study funded by Status of Women Canada, a federal agency, indicated that systemic barriers to professional licensure had not disappeared in the decade since the TFAPTO report was published. The research project, which involved over two hundred foreign-trained professionals living in Windsor, Ontario, showed that both the length of time and the excessive costs involved in recredentialing remained significant obstacles to re-entry to professional practice for new immigrants (Azuh 1998). Eighty-eight percent of those surveyed had to upgrade their skills through professional education courses, and more than 30 percent had to begin their training anew (24). Health professionals, by far the largest group surveyed, constituted nearly one-quarter of those included in the study.

The Facts Are In! A Study of the Characteristics and Experiences of Immigrants Seeking Employment in Regulated Professions in Ontario, published by the Ontario Ministry of Training, Colleges and Universities, was released in 2002. The report acknowledged that 71.1 percent of those holding professional degrees upon arrival reported having the greatest difficulty with the licensing process, considering it to be very difficult, compared with 27.3 percent of those with some professional education and 26.8 percent of those with a diploma or trade certificate, 41 percent with a bachelor's degree, 43 percent with a master's degree, and 33.3 percent with a doctorate (Ontario 2002, 29). Only 41.6 percent of professionals were employed in their exact or a related profession, while 15.3 were unemployed and 43.1 percent were in non-professional jobs (33).

On the eve of the legalization of midwifery, the Transitional Council needed to establish a process for assessing the training of those midwives who wished to become registered but who had not gained access through the Michener Institute Pre-registration Program. These included both women who had been practising in the province and who had not been admitted to or had failed the Michener Institute program, and those whose credentials were obtained outside of Ontario. A registration committee, to whom responsibility for this task had been delegated, published their recommendations on 28 June 1993. The committee consisted of long-time midwifery activist and practising midwife Elizabeth Allemang, sociologists Hugh and Pat Armstrong, and British-trained practising midwife Freda Seddon.

Using the *Access!* report as a point of reference, the registration committee recommended that the credentialing process for those with previous midwifery training use a prior learning assessment model. The report reiterated the working definition for prior learning assessment that had recently been adopted by the Prior Learning Assessment Secretariat of the Ontario Council of Regents for Colleges of Applied Arts and Technology: "Prior learning assessment [PLA] is a process using a series of tools, which assist learners to reflect, identify, recognize, articulate and demonstrate past learning in order to have it measured, compared to some standard, and in some way acknowledged by a Credentialing [sic] body. It is based on the premise that adults acquire skills and knowledge through many means of formal or informal study. For Ontario's Colleges of Applied Arts and Technology, a PLA system evaluates this learning and relates it to courses and programs for the purpose of granting college credit" (Allemang et al. 1993, 19).

There are a number of reasons that prior learning assessment made sense for the new profession. In the absence of a provincial or national credential assessment agency, the fledgling College of Midwives would have had to wait a considerable length of time and expend significant financial resources to develop a system that would rate educational equivalencies from midwifery education programs around the world. In addition to the profoundly difficult task of establishing educational equivalencies, many trained professionals, particularly those who have become refugees or political exiles, cannot easily gain access to records and transcripts. Prior learning assessment seemed the most expedient and equitable process given limited resources.

In addition, the re-emergent profession had relied on apprenticeship and non-institutional learning as its primary training model for many years, and it needed not only to validate this educational model, but to acknowledge the expertise of those practising midwives who were not grandparented into practice but who still sought registration. Although the process appeared equitable, it compelled women with many years of midwifery training and practice to undergo a long, arduous, and expensive re-assessment process.

The Prior Learning and Experience Assessment (PLEA) program of the College of Midwives of Ontario has been held up as the gold standard of equitable professional accreditation programs for foreign-trained professionals. In the *Toronto Star* series cited above, the College was credited with allowing foreign-trained midwives to have their skills assessed through objective structured clinical examinations (OSCE), a process the article claimed led to the accreditation of twenty-three out of twenty-seven applicants and that the *Star* writer sees as far more liberal than the restrictive policies applied to foreign-trained physicians in the province (Hurst 1999, A8). However, the numbers the article cites are deceiving. They in no way reflect the extraordinary rate of attrition from the PLEA process, nor do they reveal whether the process has been an equitable one for women of colour, even though the series focuses largely on the experiences of racialized-minority professionals.

The Community Advisory Committee to the PLA Project
Around the time of legalization, there was mounting evidence that immigrant midwives of colour comprised a considerable proportion of those who would seek to become registered through the Prior Learning Assessment project. By May 1994, 48 percent of the nine hundred requests for information about registration received by the College of Midwives of Ontario had come from women with midwifery training from the Philippines (25.1 percent), Jamaica (3.4 percent), Nigeria (3.4 percent), Pakistan (2.9 percent), India (2.4 percent), Hong Kong (1.9 percent), Iran (1.9 percent), Ghana (1.4 percent), China (1.4 percent), Guyana (1 percent), and Somalia (1 percent) (College of Midwives 1994a, 3). The cohort of British-trained midwives, who made up 30 percent of those seeking information, probably included a substantial percentage of women of colour.[12] Having publicly embraced an equity agenda, the Transitional Council needed to find a forum where this numerically significant group of midwives of colour could have an impact on the PLA process.

In September 1993, the Transitional Council convened a community advisory committee to the Prior Learning Assessment project. Of the twenty-two attendees, seven were women of colour. Women of colour formed a distinct minority in relation to white women at every meeting of the committee.[13] Carmencita Hernandez, a well-known community activist and founder of the Coalition of Visible Minority Women, spoke about the excitement that the PLA project had generated among immigrant midwives who hoped to practise their profession in Ontario. She proposed that Filipino women, whose inquiries to the Transitional Council had comprised the largest percentage of total calls, were willing to assist in developing a portfolio course and in collecting oral histories on the nature of midwifery practice in the Philippines.[14] Hernandez proposed that the committee needed to find ways to ensure that the early cohort of PLA graduates would include significant numbers of racialized minority women. Her concerns were echoed by Betty Wu-Lawrence, a public health nurse active in the Chinese Canadian Nurses Association, who had been appointed to the Transitional Council.

Filipino midwives took an exceedingly proactive stance in relationship to the Prior Learning Assessment project. In November of 1993, the National Council of Canadian Filipino Associations invited trained Filipino midwives to a discussion of midwifery regulation with members of the Transitional Council. Eighteen out of the twenty Philippines-trained midwives who had contacted the Transitional Council's offices about accreditation in Ontario attended the meeting ("Regulating Midwifery," 1993). In a strategy session following the meeting, those attending articulated the barriers to practice that they felt would impede the entrance of Filipino midwives to the midwifery profession. First, the group acknowledged that a significant percentage of credentialed midwives worked as nannies and that for this group, taking time off work for training was simply impossible. They also recognized that the proposed fee of $2,500 was well beyond the means of many of the women represented in the group. In addition, the immigration status of some midwives as live-in caregivers guaranteed at least a two-year gap in practice, a deficit that would put them at a disadvantage in an accreditation process that promised advanced standing to those with recent practice experience. The group proposed the formation of an organization whose goals would include lobbying for equitable access to the profession, looking for funding for training and professional review sessions, and initiating a bursary fund for those seeking registration (National Council of Canadian Filipino Organizations 1994, 10).

The organization that emerged from the strategy session was the Association of Philippine Midwives. One of the group's stated purposes was to "liaise with similar organizations and with the College of Midwives of Ontario" (National Council of Filipino Canadian Associations 1994, 8). In the summer of 1994, the group presented a formal proposal to the College of Midwives in which it outlined a plan to organize a series of workshops to "heighten awareness among foreign-trained midwives in the immigrant and racial minority communities on the history of the practice of Midwifery in

Ontario," and to "provide support and/or networking capabilities to foreign-trained midwives."[15] The project organizers proposed a budget of $6,500 and pledged a community contribution of $3,000; nevertheless, the College of Midwives denied the group funding.[16]

One woman who helped to formulate the funding proposal expressed her disappointment with the College's failure to support the effort: "But I was really hopeful that the women, the regulatory body, would be more open and acceptable. Just like you think there might be solidarity in terms of women. And also in terms of issues related to women ... I felt that it was not maximized. They had the power to do something. Thirty-five hundred dollars is no big amount" (Interview no. 30). Discourses of female unity across other axes of difference – the midwifery project's stock in trade – had underpinned Filipino midwives' understanding of the movement for legalization and had created expectations of solidarity that were unfulfilled. The woman quoted above, a participant in the Transitional Council/College of Midwives' community advisory council on the PLA process, felt that she and others had had no influence on policy, partly because they were outsiders and partly because their primary loyalty was, unsurprisingly, not to the midwifery movement but to the achievement of employment equity for Filipino midwives. She explained the constraints on her participation: "I know it's difficult to influence policy unless you're inside, right? And unless you know the steps to go about it ... My goal wasn't for *them*" (Interview no. 30).

One policy area immigrant midwives involved in the community advisory council did attempt to influence was language testing. The Task Force on Access to Professions and Trades in Ontario had flagged language testing as a key barrier. "Emphasis on training in general fluency rather than on occupation-specific proficiency development" argued the report, had made it difficult for some professionals to achieve accreditation (TFAPTO 1989, xv). At their 1993 meeting with Transitional Council members, Filipino midwives echoed the TFAPTO *Access!* report in flagging the inequity of the TOEFL (Test of English as a Foreign Language) exam used to measure English language skills ("Regulating Midwifery" 1993). The Transitional Council's response was to develop a profession-specific language exam that was piloted in June 1994. The College's decision to offer no exemptions from the language exam, even for native English speakers, was conveyed to the community advisory committee by CMO council member Brenda Hyatali at their 20 June 1994 meeting. Objections were raised by several women of colour at the 20 September 1994 meeting and at the next meeting on 1 November 1994. Narinder Kainth, representing the Scarborough Grace Birthing Centre, expressed her own opposition and stated that there had not been support for the policy on the community advisory council. Prior Learning Assessment project coordinator Diane Pudas dismissed the issue, claiming that no objections had been raised when the decision had been announced in June.[17] Both the interviews conducted for this study and statistics about participation in the PLA process demonstrate that language testing has been a significant roadblock both to midwives who are native English speakers and to those for whom English is a second or third language.

The implementation by the CMO of a major policy that was clearly opposed by immigrant women serving on the community advisory committee bespeaks the token nature of this committee. Despite the lack of heed paid to their opinions, the support of immigrant women of colour became an important resource in the College's bid to win funding from the Access to Professions and Trades Demonstration Project Fund for the next phase of PLA: the "multifaceted assessment" of midwifery skills. PLA project coordinator Diane Pudas had sent a memo in April 1994 in which she informed registration committee members that the provincial government's Access to Professions and Trades Unit had, in a conversation with her, emphasized their equity mandate. Therefore, she concluded, "It would appear to be to our advantage to solicit co-sponsorship from community groups that have members that wish to apply to the CMO for registration." The College of Midwives' successful funding proposal claimed that "the needs of immigrant women to access the profession of midwifery coincide with Ontario's need for accessible midwifery care" (CMO 1994a, 3). Groups such as the Caribbean midwives group, the Filipino Midwives Association, the Chinese Canadian Nurses Association, and the Coalition of Visible Minority Women wrote enthusiastic letters of support. However, as with the equity committee initiative, consultations with marginalized groups produced benefit for the midwifery project but seemed to produce little in the way of access to the profession for immigrant midwives of colour.

The Prior Learning Assessment project was launched in October 1994 with three public orientation sessions that had been widely advertised across the province. Of the nearly one thousand women who had inquired about access to practice, only 337 actually attended these sessions, which cost each participant ten dollars. The orientation was considered the first step in the PLA process and introduced potential applicants to the multi-tiered process. The first major requirement was a two-part profession-specific language exam, after the successful completion of which the candidate was to submit a four-part portfolio that included a clinical practice equivalency portfolio, an autobiographical portfolio, a baccalaureate equivalency portfolio, and a core competency portfolio. For admission to the PLA process, midwives needed to be either graduates of a recognized midwifery program or registered to practise in another jurisdiction and have a minimum clinical experience of attendance at no fewer than forty births, twenty of which must have been as primary midwife (assuming sole responsibility for the parturient woman in the intrapartum period). Alternatively, applicants were to have attended forty births as a primary midwife or at least thirty as a primary midwife and twenty as an assistant to the primary midwife (CMO 1994b).

The admission criteria were designed to include both those Ontario midwives who had not graduated from the Michener Institute program, as well as midwives trained outside of Canada in institutional midwifery education programs. Nearly 50 percent of those who applied to the first cycle of PLA were from the latter category. The first cycle of the Prior Learning Assessment process had a rather dramatic rate of attrition. As was mentioned above, only 337 of the thousand women who expressed interest in the process actually attended the first orientation. Of these, 165 submitted applications to the College. Only 126 of this group took the first language examination, late in 1994. Nearly half of the applicants failed that exam and only sixty-three went on to take the second half. Fifty-six of these submitted portfolios to the College and fifty-one went on to undergo the multifaceted assessment process. Candidates whose baccalaureate credentials were considered outdated (older than ten years for sciences, older than fifteen years for social sciences) were required to sit "challenge" exams or re-enrol in equivalency courses. Most candidates were required to enrol in a course entitled "Midwifery in Ontario" that had not been part of the original PLA plan. Initially scheduled to grant eligibility to successful candidates in the summer of 1995, the first PLA cycle took nearly four years. Of the twenty-seven who were eligible, only seventeen of the original 165 applicants were registered as of May 1998. In October 1997, forty women, including eleven returning candidates from cycle one, embarked on a slightly modified second PLEA cycle.[18] Half of cycle one candidates were white women who had practised previous to legislation in Ontario. Only 2 percent of the second cycle's candidates fit that description.[19]

By May 1998, the percentage of women of colour among registered midwives in the province bore little resemblance to the percentage who originally expressed interest in qualifying to practise. In December 1994 there was just one registered midwife of colour out of the sixty-eight who had completed the Michener Institute program. By 1998, out of 126 registered midwives, twelve were women of colour and one was an Aboriginal woman; an additional nineteen women of colour were scheduled to complete the Prior Learning and Experience Assessment program. By July 2000, approximately nineteen women out of 180 registered midwives were identified as women of colour or Aboriginal women, but not all had succeeded in securing employment in the province. Only about half of these women entered midwifery practice through the Prior Learning and Experience Assessment route. As was noted in the Introduction, today, women of colour represent about 12 percent of the province's nearly three hundred currently practising midwives.

Language Proficiency and Cost: Two Barriers to Participation

Two of the most salient barriers to equitable access in the Prior Learning Assessment process were the language exams and the cost. In both the first and second cycles of the Prior Learning Assessment process, more than half of those who submitted applications failed the program's first step, the profession-specific language exam. Given that a very large percentage of applicants were from countries in the South where English is not the dominant language, it is highly likely that the bulk of those who failed the language exam were women of colour.[20] And, while the confidentiality of the College of Midwives' exam precludes any detailed analysis of possible cultural bias or other exclusionary functions of the exam, those interviewed, among them native English speakers, questioned the level of English skills required to pass the exam. They referred to technical aspects of the exam, such as the speed of the audio tape.[21] They also asked why the ability to interpret highly local sociocultural expressions seemed to be part of the assessment process.[22] Some midwives I interviewed even questioned the language assessment procedures, pointing out that in a province as multicultural as Ontario, no concomitant process evaluates "Canadian" midwives' competency in any of the non-dominant languages spoken in Ontario. One interviewee, a native English speaker and long-time resident of Canada, explained her own struggles with the taped part of the exam and mentioned the difficulties someone less skilled than she might experience in interpreting dominant linguistic and cultural signs. Naming the speaker on the tape as "Canadian," this midwife emphasized the culture-bound nature of the exam content, neatly unmasking dominance masquerading as invisibility. "The second [part] was this Canadian person talking fast on a tape," she recalled, "... and at the end they'll ask you, 'Is this woman happy or sad?' Well, no·not really like that but, 'What did you understand? What were they saying?' It was too fast. I passed the test but it was too fast. So I'm sure that people not familiar with this Canadian accent are going to miss the under thing. And it's a psychological question where you have to decide, what does it really say" (Interview no. 13).

Key midwifery spokespeople and activists have communicated to the public that the "culturally sensitive practice of midwifery" is fundamental to the profession's philosophy (Ontario IRCM 1994, 86). The need to provide educational programs and labour support for birthing women in their native languages has been touted as a fundamental element of such culturally sensitive care. However, the College of Midwives' practices around language suggest a different reality. By narrowing rather than expanding the linguistic resources of the province's midwives, exclusion related to language reflects what Ella Shohat and Robert Stam (1994, 193) have defined as "linguistic non-reciprocity": the demand that subordinate groups speak the dominant language but that no reciprocal requirement to acquire communicative resources is imposed on dominant linguistic groups. Moreover, exclusionary language exams and high failure rates reinscribe foreign-trained professionals as lacking competencies seen as fundamental to "Canadianness." As Eve Haque (1999, 5) points out, focusing on language competency "establishes the cultural lack in the immigrant, thus making it impossible to consider any other framework that might locate the lack elsewhere, for example, the lack being in defining the Canadian nation state as only bilingual and only in two European languages, no less."

Policies that privilege dominant language groups are part of larger disciplinary practices serving to differentiate not only between those who belong in the nation's most prosperous and prestigious occupational groups and those who do not, but between those who belong in the nation and those who do not (Tollefson 1991). Requiring English language testing not only for those who were not native speakers of English but for native speakers as well – a policy formulated by the College of Midwives to avoid charges of discrimination – served to remind native English-speaking midwives of colour from former English colonies of their outsider status in the profession and the nation. Many of those interviewed expressed anger about being made to spend hundreds of dollars on the examinations when they had been raised and educated and had worked for years in the English language.

In midwifery, the languages of postcolonial subjects both disprove the unity of the nation and present an audible disruption to the claims to respectability of a profession labouring to overturn a century of inferiorizing narratives about midwives, some of which have relied on racist and xenophobic discourses. One strategy for interrupting this dynamic would be to recognize the critical value of communicative skills in languages other than English and to reward, rather than punish, those who possess them. A secondary strategy would involve providing supportive educational settings for acquiring the dominant linguistic and sociocultural knowledge necessary for economic survival. In her article on equitable assessment of the oral English of foreign-trained teachers of English in Australia, Rosemary Viete (1998) has argued that the ability to communicate in a given language and to function successfully in the sociocultural context in which that language is embedded can only be assessed fairly if the person examined has been provided, prior to the examination, with significant support in gaining such competency. While there was one notably unsuccessful attempt at this – the establishment of a collaborative mentorship program for midwives with Chinese language skills – it was only recently that a bridging program put in place by the College of Midwives began to offer occupation-specific language training that can be taken prior to the required Midwifery Language Proficiency Test.[23] For those women attempting to become registered midwives in the first and second cycles of the PLA/PLEA project, the language exams reproduced employment inequality in the province by barring the way of those otherwise competent midwives who failed the English language exams.

The cost of completing the Prior Learning Assessment/Prior Learning and Experience Assessment process constituted another significant exclusionary policy. Course fees, textbooks, child care, room and board, and stipends were freely provided to those practising midwives who participated in the Michener Institute's midwifery integration project, whereas the PLA/PLEA process was run entirely on a cost-recovery basis. The cost to participants in the first cycle was $2,400 for all aspects of assessment by the College of Midwives. If the candidate was deemed to be lacking baccalaureate credits, she had to write a challenge exam or pursue the more lengthy and expensive process of completing a university-level course. Like those who attended the Michener Institute program, PLA candidates incurred child care and travel expenses and experienced loss of income when attending full-time courses such as "Midwifery in Ontario." They also incurred costs for obtaining, copying, notarizing, and transporting documentation of their professional experience and education. My own interview data, as well as recent statistical information on inequitable earning patterns between European and non-European immigrants (Tran 2004; Galabuzi 2001; Lian and Matthews 1998; Ornstein 1996), indicate that exceedingly high recertification costs worked to keep immigrant midwives of colour from participating in the College of Midwives Prior Learning Assessment and Prior Learning and Experience Assessment programs.

The second cycle began during spring 1997 and was renamed "Prior Learning and Experience Assessment" (PLEA). This cycle cost candidates over $600 more than its predecessor. For those who were able sit the baccalaureate challenge exams, the cost of challenging all five university-level courses was $775. For those who actually needed to enrol in and pass the requisite baccalaureate courses, the tuition costs were often as high as $700 per course. One candidate, who was close to finishing at the time of our interview, estimated that the cost of her recertification in a profession in which she already had training and in which she had successfully practised was close to $8,000 (Interview no. 7). And while many needed extra assistance to make their way through the maze of portfolio preparation and other challenges, few of those interviewed could afford to pay the fee ($100 per course) for a series of five one-day preparatory seminars designed by the College to introduce candidates to the PLEA process.

Cost creates exclusion when income is inequitably distributed among racialized groups in society. Analyses of data from the 1991 census indicate that while there were significant differences among groups and within groups, non-European ethnoracial groups in the Metropolitan Toronto area had mean incomes which were between $6,000 and $12,000 below the city-wide mean annual employment income of $31,300 (Ornstein 1996, 8-9). Between 1996 and 1998, there was a 24 percent gap in average before-tax income and a 20 percent gap in after-tax income between racialized group members and other Canadians (Galabuzi 2001). A recently published Canada-wide study that controlled for multiple variables including gender, age, age squared, marital status, province of residence, metropolitan versus non-metropolitan area of residence, geographic mobility in the past five years, period of immigration, knowledge of official languages, occupational level, industrial sector, weeks worked and weeks worked squared, and full- versus part-time weeks worked concluded that wage inequity along racial lines was present at every educational and occupational level (Lian and Matthews 1998). Although comparable data are not yet available for the 2001 census, preliminary analyses indicate that the racial gap in earnings has actually deepened (McIsaac 2003, 61).

Analyses of the 1996 Canadian census also show significant discrepancies between the earnings of recent immigrant women of colour and recent white female immigrants, with women of colour earning on average $16,300 and white women earning $20,100 (MacKinnon 1999, B1). In Toronto, where the vast majority of people of colour in the province reside, not only do recently immigrated women of colour earn lower salaries, 21 percent of such women in the age category of twenty-five to forty-four years old are unemployed as opposed to 6 percent of their white counterparts (Badets and Howatson-Leo 1999). In the absence of provincial subsidies for the PLA/PLEA process, and given the lack of provision for loans or bursaries for those undergoing it, high recertification costs pose an unfair barrier to those whose incomes fall below the national mean due to systemic racism.

Bureaucracy and Systemic Racism

Administrative delays and errors were endemic to both the first and second cycles of the PLA/PLEA, and played a role, I believe, in producing exclusionary outcomes. Eight out of ten immigrant midwives of colour interviewed who participated in the PLA/PLEA process described being frustrated with the College's delayed or non-existent response to requests for information and/or the curt manner or short time frame in which payment for various parts of the process was requested. One woman reported that after inquiring for over a year about the status of her application – which included irreplaceable original documents retrieved from her politically volatile homeland – she was informed that it had been lost. She did not reapply (Interview no. 9). Many of these women described the tenacity required to gain access to information about participating in the process. One woman explained that when she phoned the College, she inevitably got an answering machine. "I left my message, left my message, left my message; nobody returned my call" (Interview no. 3). Another woman who had asked to be alerted when the first PLA process started, but who never was, placed regular, insistent phone calls to the College about the process's second phase. Despite having given the College her name and mailing address several times, she received no information. In the course of yet another telephone inquiry, she was asked to give her name and address yet again, after which information began to arrive. After a year of frustrating contacts with the College, this immigrant midwife of colour felt that "the whole process ... I just find is just very ... is a process I feel is there to discourage people. It's one that is there to weigh you down ... There are a lot of things that could be done differently to make the process run a lot smoother, which, if they claim to be as professional, as on the ball, and as fair as they say they want to make it ... It's not a fair process at all, I don't believe. I just don't feel it to be a fair process" (Interview no. 7).

The College explained away the mistakes by claiming that there was inadequate staffing and by using the "heroic myth" of midwifery's re-emergence to deflect blame. One immigrant midwife of colour remembers being told that "they were just three [staff] and the huge things that they did, and 'til now [midwives had] sacrificed their own personal life to reach this" (Interview no. 9). Another applicant was told that "resources are limited and we have to put them toward the midwives and the PLEA candidates" (Interview no. 7). We should regard these practices as neither random nor benign. The allocation of inadequate resources to the PLA/PLEA process must be seen as indicative of the low priority assigned either by the College of Midwives or the province, or by both, to the incorporation into the profession of previously practising midwives, many of whom were women of colour. Midwifery representatives had successfully negotiated ample, if not lavish, resources for the integration of practising midwives through the Michener Institute program, but their negotiating skills had obviously not been employed to create the conditions by which foreign-trained non-practising midwives could re-enter the profession for which they had been trained.

A 1985 study conducted by the Urban Alliance on Race Relations and the Toronto Social Planning Council found significant evidence of discrimination by employers against researchers posing as job seekers using non-European names and/or speaking with non-dominant accents (Henry and Ginzberg 1985). White Canadian researchers were told in response to telephone inquiries that jobs were already filled in only 13 percent of cases; white immigrants were told this in 31 percent of cases; black West Indians were told jobs were closed in 36 percent of cases; and Indo-Pakistani researchers were told this in nearly 44 percent of cases (5). Nearly two decades later racialized individuals continue to encounter discrimination. A Statistics Canada study of ethnic diversity published in 2002 reported that "about 20% of visible minorities or 587,000 people said they had sometimes or often experienced discrimination or unfair treatment in the previous five years because of their ethnicity, culture, race, skin colour, language, accent or religion" (Statistics Canada 2002, 21). Fifty-six percent of those who had sometimes or often experienced discrimination because of their ethnocultural characteristics reported that their experiences of discriminatory treatment most often occurred at work or when applying for employment (24).

There may be many explanations for the high rate of attrition from the Prior Learning Assessment process by foreign-trained midwives. One such possible explanation is that some were deterred by the College's constant deferrals and bureaucratic bungles. Perhaps not intentionally racist, these occurrences may have produced racist effects when experienced by racialized "others," whose encounters with white gatekeepers have reinforced the message that access to the nation's rewards are not theirs for the taking.

This chapter has documented the numerous ways that Ontario midwifery has been maintained as a "white space," despite the presence in the province of scores of trained midwives of colour. Fundamental to practices of racist exclusion has been the understanding that midwifery is a project formulated to address gender oppression and that women are positioned in the social matrix in a uniformly subordinate way, rather than in a hierarchical fashion. Such an understanding has rendered race a largely irrelevant consideration in the formulation of policies and in everyday practices related to midwifery's re-emergence. Many structural factors, including the threat of professional or legal reprisals, created conditions in which women of colour may have feared practising in the quasi-legal atmosphere that characterized the early years of midwifery's consolidation as an alternative health care practice. However, there existed ample evidence during midwifery's formative period that women of colour with midwifery skills and philosophies of care congruent with local practices wished fervently to practise their profession. Uninspired attempts at inclusion did nothing to increase the participation of women of colour in the midwifery movement and later served to reinscribe marginalized women's identities while simultaneously producing white midwives as benevolent. Government-appointed bodies remained unrepresentative of the large number of midwives of colour in the province and enacted numerous policies that created roadblocks to the entry of midwives of colour to professional practice. Seeing their project as one that addressed the "universal needs of women" allowed white midwives and their supporters to rationalize exclusionary measures. All the while, they consolidated white solidarity in the profession, left intact a history of racist exclusion in the health care field, and reinforced racial segmentation in a province significantly populated by people of colour. The same unexamined belief in universal sisterhood propelled Ontario midwives to travel to Third World sites and border spaces where significant material and discursive rewards were made available to them through access to the bodies of subaltern mothers.

3
Midwifery Tourism

> With all tourist sites, commerce depends on the construction of a desirable Other – often one that titillates as well as appeals – capable of attracting outsiders. This construction can create inequitable interactions between local and traveler that actually serve to reinforce disparity while being represented as mutually beneficial. In these international interactions ... the flow from center to periphery, from here to there, is virtually unidirectional ... The disparity of interactions can be charted in this flow: when "they" come "here," we educate them; when "we" go "there," they service us.
>
> – Ryan Bishop and Lillian Robinson, *Night Market*

In the course of conducting this research, I discovered that a significant number of Ontario midwives had acquired training and experience in Third World maternity clinics. Many, but not all, travelled to garner the requisite quota of births for participation in the Michener Institute program designed to integrate practising midwives into the health care system. Whether birth numbers were required or not, the experience obtained in these clinics enhanced the midwives' professional status, enabling them to claim first-hand knowledge of the birth practices of Third World women, a commodity valued highly both in the medical and the alternative birth communities. This practice continues today, as aspiring midwives, midwifery students, and practising midwives continue to seek expertise in these sites. It seemed profoundly ironic that while immigrant midwives of colour were largely unable to use their professional expertise in Ontario, practice experience acquired in the Third World enabled white Ontario midwives to qualify for registration in the province. That Ontario midwives derived substantial material benefit from their encounters with Third World women seemed to confirm

recent scholarly claims that both nineteenth- and twentieth-century feminist projects in the West have been contingent upon global conditions of
imperialism and racial dominance (Burton 1994; Chaudhuri and Strobel
1992; Grewal 1996; Mohanty 1991; Pierson and Chaudhuri 1999; Pratt 1992;
Ware 1992). This chapter looks at some of the transnational processes that
have made birthing women's bodies in the Third World available for the
educational consumption and material advantage of First World women. I
describe the global conditions that make this travel possible and analyze
some of the travelogues I have gathered from "midwifery tourists." These
travelogues recount violence and benevolence, as well as innocence and
complicity, but, above all, they demonstrate how feminist projects that rely
on unexamined notions of "global sisterhood" actually reproduce unequal
relations of power between women.

Crossing the Border for Midwifery Experience

While some Ontario midwives acquired formal midwifery credentials abroad,
most learned the profession through intensive self-study and apprenticeship. However, opportunities to gain and exercise a broad spectrum of clinical skills were rather limited in the period prior to proclamation of midwifery
legislation. Barred from practising in hospitals, midwives could employ their
full expertise only at home births. The twenty-six midwives who were practising in Toronto, for example, attended, between 1983 and 1988, the home
births of 1001 women, which meant that in a period critical to the establishment of midwifery's credibility, a Toronto midwife had, *on average*, complete
professional responsibility for fewer than eight births per year (Tyson 1991).[1]
Obtaining clinical experience became a matter of some import for women
who wished to devote their professional lives to the practice of midwifery.

For midwives practising in the legal limbo that characterized the prelegislation period, obtaining wider clinical experience was crucial to gaining public confidence in the viability of midwifery care and to stemming
physician opposition to the burgeoning practice. Such experience took on
even greater significance with the advent of legislation, when it became a
basic requirement for licensure. In 1986 the Ontario government accepted
a recommendation of the Health Professions Legislation Review that midwifery become a regulated profession and appointed a provincial task force
to develop implementation strategies. The Task Force on the Implementation of Midwifery in Ontario made clear in its recommendations that attendance at a substantial number of births would be required of currently
practising midwives seeking to be grandparented into practice.

Responding to the need for its members to acquire maximum clinical
experience in the minimum time possible, the midwives' professional organization, the Association of Ontario Midwives, scrambled to find clinical

sites where midwives could gain experience. Lacking institutional midwifery credentials, most Ontario midwives had no access to American or European clinical settings where midwifery was the standard of care. And while some midwives found placements in rural areas in the Philippines and in Guatemala, Haiti, or Jamaica, the vast majority of those who travelled enrolled as interns at independent midwifery clinics on the US-Mexico border, a geopolitical space where, in the words of Norma Alarcon (1996, 45), "the third world rubs against the first." For a fee, Ontario midwives could receive didactic training and attend Mexican women who, for a variety of reasons, discussed below, crossed to the United States to deliver their babies. An Ontario midwife who spent time at one such clinic in the late 1970s was able to name more than twenty colleagues who had also done so in the years prior to legislation. For these women, Canadian nationality and white skin served as passports to unobstructed border crossing and instant authority in the border spaces made available to them through this "midwifery tourism."[2]

Travel and the Female Subject of Modernity
As postcolonial theorist Lata Mani (1998, 3) has observed, colonized space has frequently served as a "theater of social experimentation" wherein Europeans have sought to critique and reconfigure the social relations of "home." In the previous two centuries, European women's ventures into such space have allowed them to claim social identities unavailable to them under Western patriarchies. This area of inquiry has been a fruitful one, with feminist/postcolonial historians and theorists crafting a burgeoning "cultural retrospection of empire" (Ware 1992, 229) aimed at untangling European women's role in the establishment and consolidation of imperial rule. In colonized locales, Western women were frequently able to act outside the restrictive gender roles available at home because cross-gender bonds of race in the colonies were far more important to maintaining colonial hierarchies than was upholding the gendered social organization of the imperial metropolis.

Scholarship exploring the historical relationship between feminism and imperialism can be useful in understanding contemporary social relations because the contours of the imperial world and the very categories and spatial boundaries that it created and policed continue to hold sway (Razack 1998a). Barbara Heron's study (1999, 186) demonstrated how white Canadian women who participate in overseas development work are able to enjoy a "release from the strictured constructions of white femininity" within largely male-dominated development projects. "Faced with the numerically overwhelming physical presence of the Other," Heron explains, "[the] response of whiteness seems to entail extending a degree of insider status and white power relations to women development workers albeit in gender specific ways." Heron's interview subjects emerged from their development experiences with a "new narrative of self" (189) reflecting a subjectivity approximating that of the modern bourgeois subject: free, unfettered, and able to act in the world in ways unrestrained by hierarchical gender norms. Like that achieved by their historical counterparts, this contemporary feminist recoding of the self accomplished by development workers and other white female travellers, such as Ontario midwives, requires (and subsequently reproduces) the colonial context.

Why "Midwifery Tourism"?

"Tourism" rather than "travel" best characterizes the process by which white women from Ontario engaged in encounters with providers and consumers of birthing care on the US-Mexico border. The term "travel," as Inderpal Grewal (1996, 2) has noted, implies a "universal form of mobility" and consequently elides contemporary forms of population movement that are inherently coercive: the results of war, interethnic conflict, forced migration, and the movement of people seeking reprieve from the decimation of social and economic structures wrought by policies of structural adjustment. "Tourism," on the other hand, connotes a largely voluntary form of travel available to those whose citizenship status and financial resources permit them access to locations and populations deemed desirable.

An appetite for the exotic has long fuelled the modern tourism enterprise. Some of its newest forms claim to offer the tourist something more morally uplifting than the pursuit of pleasure through the consumption of difference. In a context of widespread anxiety in the West around social degeneracy and planetary decline, initiatives such as ecotourism and cultural tourism promise the Western tourist access to those spaces not yet destroyed by capitalism's excesses. Indigenous cultures are fantasized in this schema as the repositories of health and wholeness, and both land and people, represented via a "revitalized primitivist stereotype," become seductive objects for tourist consumption (Jacobs 1996, 142). These forms of tourism promise a fundamental transformation of self in which the tourist's implication within neocolonial relations of power are rendered moot and these tourisms are construed as an inherently ethical and mutually beneficial engagement with the "other."

This desire for the "other" in midwifery tourism is driven by a desire for a very specific "other": the Third World mother, mythologized widely within natural-childbirth discourse as possessing innate feminine birthing knowledge as yet uncorrupted by Western medical practices. From American anthropologist Margaret Mead in the 1940s, to British childbirth reformer Sheila Kitzinger in the 1990s, primitive subjects have been deployed to decry the impaired childbearing capacities of women in the West (Mead 1967; Kitzinger 1992).

Indigenous Latin American women have been awarded a particularly revered status in natural childbirth iconography. Bridget Jordan's *Birth in Four Cultures*, a scholarly ethnography of childbearing (1983, 40) "with the assistance family and friends" among Maya Indians in Yucatan, Mexico – a book once impossible to find – is currently in its fourth printing, having been used widely, by the author's admission, "in the ongoing enterprise of changing the American way of birth" (Jordan quoted in Davis-Floyd and Sargent 1997, 1). For many years, *Birth*, a medical journal devoted to the reform of clinical maternity care practices, has featured Latin American birth art, from reproductions of Mixtec genealogical-historical manuscripts to a contemporary painting entitled *Homage to the Mothers of Latin America*. In Canada, the image of a Nicaraguan *partera* (midwife) is emblazoned on a poster promoting the Association of Ontario Midwives, and a film produced in 1979 in a Brazilian hospital is still enthusiastically screened more than twenty years later. The theme is that childbearing women in the West have lost the innate ability to birth naturally, while those in the Third World, frozen in time, have retained it.[3] Indigenous Latin American childbearing women can be constructed as particularly authentic through links to iconographic figures such as Quiché Indian activist Rigoberta Menchu, as well as through popular representations of the forest-dwelling suppliers of raw materials to The Body Shop, who are touted as having access to the secrets of natural health through substances unknown in the West.

Midwifery tourism is a material practice involving travel from one place to another, the exchange of money, the performance of medical acts, and the issuing of certificates of completion. However, it is also inextricably interwoven with, and produced by, discursive constructs. A discourse of authenticity makes the Third World woman a desirable object of engagement because she is a "full representative of ... her tradition" (Spivak 1999, 60). However, it is the discourse of global sisterhood that allows midwifery tourists to deflect any implication in the North/South relations of global inequality. As one midwife told me about her experience on the US-Mexico border, "There was something that went beyond borders, in terms of midwifery care and terms of caring for each other as women. It was such a common bond that it didn't matter who you were at that point ... I felt you were just 'with woman' and all you had to be was a woman to make that happen" (Interview no. 21). Framed within discourses of borderlessness and benevolence, midwifery tourism allowed Canadian women to produce themselves as respectable professionals and to rationalize both the specific relations of violence experienced in the border clinics and the global violence that produces the geopolitical spaces in which those clinics have thrived.

The US-Mexico Border as Transnational Space

The US-Mexico border is a space characterized by histories of colonial conquest, dramatic demographic shifts, and aggressive economic incursions by multinational corporations. In the words of Chicana theorist Gloria Anzaldua (1987, 2), the border is a "1,950 mile open wound." The proliferation since 1965 of scores of maquiladoras, or export-processing factories, which are largely American- or Japanese-owned, has dramatically altered the population of northern Mexico, drawing steadily northward residents of central and southern Mexican states to border regions such as Matamoros/Reynosa, Ciudad Juárez/El Paso, Calexico/Mexicali, and San Diego/Tijuana. Factories employ Mexican workers at low wages – typically the peso equivalent of between US$40 and US$50 per month – which are inadequate to support an individual worker, much less an entire family (Salzinger 2003, 138). The largest concentration of maquiladora workers in Mexico is in Ciudad Juárez, which borders El Paso, Texas. These workers, Debbie Nathan (1999, 27) explains, put in "forty-eight hour weeks soldering electronics boards, plugging wires into car dashboards, binding surgical gowns and sorting millions of cosmetics discount coupons mailed by North Americans to P.O. boxes in El Paso." In the Matamoros/Reynosa maquiladoras, the organization of work has been described as "reminiscent of 19th century US sweatshops ... Tayloristic and authoritarian, with detailed division of labor, repetitive simple tasks and piecework wages" (Moure-Eraso, 1997, 597). Mexican labour from this border space makes possible the consumption of inexpensive consumer goods and other commodities that contribute to the high standard of living in the West.

As elsewhere in the globalized economy, employment in the maquiladoras has a distinctly gendered dimension. The proliferation of export-processing plants in free-trade zones around the globe has created unprecedented employment opportunities for women, who are considered to be a dexterous, docile, apolitical, and endlessly replaceable workforce. While as recently as a decade ago, 75 to 85 percent of Ciudad Juárez's maquiladora workers were women, this number has been reduced in recent years to around 50 percent of the total workforce. Not only has increasing militancy by female workers rendered their employment less desirable to the managers of export-processing plants, the devaluation of the peso has reduced the cost of labour, making maquila production even more profitable for transnational corporations, and the recruitment of male labour a practical necessity.[4] For the young women who do enter the maquiladora workforce, hiring is conditional on a negative pregnancy test and pregnant workers can be summarily dismissed. Employee turnover is exceedingly high and most workers have less than one year's seniority on the job (Salzinger 2003, 61). For women displaced to the north of Mexico who are unable to sustain employment in maquiladoras, domestic labour across the border offers a viable employment option. In El Paso, Texas, between eighteen thousand and twenty-six thousand homes hire domestic help, and the majority of these workers are women from Ciudad Juárez who are employed as either daily maids or live-in household workers (Wu 1998, 3). At both the personal and the global level, Third World women's labour translates into First World privilege.

Undocumented Mexican migrants are increasingly the targets of border surveillance and the objects of a strengthening discourse in the United States about the drain on the public purse (Kearney 1991). Unwanted as citizens, Mexican residents and migrants are indispensable as transnational consumers. Border cities like El Paso are economically dependent on Mexican shoppers who spend US$22 billion a year in American border cities, generating some four hundred thousand jobs and paying US$1.7 billion in taxes (Brown 1997, 105). By some estimates, nearly six thousand medical service jobs in El Paso are underwritten by Mexican nationals willing to pay for medical services, including prenatal, intrapartum, and postpartum care delivered by direct-entry midwives in out-of-hospital birth centres on the US-Mexico border (Brown 1997, 108).

White midwives and Mexican women are at the nexus of several transnational processes. Largely impoverished and displaced to the North by the promise of employment in export-processing plants, Mexican women who become pregnant require cheap and competent perinatal care. Poor or inaccessible services on the Mexican side of the border and tightened controls over services to undocumented migrants on the American side of the border (coupled with fears of deportation if they seek care in state-funded institutions) prompt some Mexican women to deliver their babies in out-of-hospital clinics run predominantly by Anglo direct-entry midwives. More than just a cheap or convenient individual solution, for these women giving birth in the United States is fundamentally an act of resistance that challenges arbitrary border delineations and creates a transnational Hispanic community through their children's right to US citizenship (Rodriguez 1996, 21; Pope 2001). A widespread practice, cross-border childbirth has gained the attention of public-health researchers hoping to improve maternal-infant health status on both sides of the border. At least two studies have shown that approximately 10 percent of border-dwelling Mexican women cross into the United States to deliver their babies, frequently without having received prenatal care (Guendelman and Jasis 1992, 10). While some of these women give birth attended by nurse-midwives in church-funded Catholic maternity homes, many receive care from direct-entry midwives (Boyer 1992). While only 0.3 percent of all births in the United States (approximately twelve thousand births) are attended by lay or direct-entry midwives, 75 percent of these are conducted in birth centres located on the US-Mexico border and the majority involve Mexican or Mexican-American women as clients (Rooks 1997, 153). "The great demand for this service," boasts one clinic's promotional pamphlet for potential students, has resulted in El Paso becoming "the heart of midwifery in the United States" (Maternidad n.d.).

Border Clinics and Tourist Schemes

The proliferation of midwifery clinics on the US-Mexico border is largely contemporaneous with the installation by transnational capitalist enterprise of export-processing industries in the north of Mexico (McCallum 1979). While numerous alternative midwifery training schemes have arisen in North America since the early 1970s, most direct-entry midwifery training has been based on attendance at home births which, according to available statistics, did not, in the last decade, exceed 0.7 percent of total births in the United States (Rooks 1997, 150). Border clinics have, for the last twenty years, been a significant training site for those unwilling or unable to pursue long and expensive apprenticeships in the few available programs. The clinics have been popular because they enable direct-entry midwifery students to attend large numbers of births within a relatively short time.[5] More recently, self-study programs have offered direct-entry midwifery students short-term "externships," primarily to impoverished Jamaican hospitals, but also to American-run birth clinics in the Philippines and Guatemala where students can garner the requisite number of births to acquire the designation "certified professional midwife" granted by the independent Midwifery Education Accreditation Council (Rooks 1997, 268). Both the border clinics and the travel schemes are contingent on transnational processes that make Third World women's bodies available for First World women's educational and professional needs.

Seven practising and non-practising white midwives or midwifery students whom I interviewed participated in midwifery tourism between 1978 and 1997. The women provided rich data on their experiences in a number of settings, including four US-Mexico border midwifery clinics. Interview subjects also provided access to clinics' promotional literature and other materials. In addition, Internet research has yielded information (including advertising materials that specifically target Canadian midwives) about travel schemes to Jamaican hospitals as well as to independent birth clinics in Guatemala, India, and the Philippines. The training programs last from eight days (a hospital stint in Jamaica) to fifteen months (a missionary midwifery training program in the Philippines). Costs vary from US$1,850 for the shortest trip to more than US$12,000 for the training program in the Philippines, with a popular three-month internship at one Texas midwifery clinic, costing US$3,750. Internships at the border clinics typically involve classroom instruction and immediate hands-on experience. Most border clinics do not require previous midwifery experience, and yet students can expect to attend twenty-five to thirty-five births in a three-month period. The Jamaican trips offer a much higher volume of births, and prospective students, according to one information letter, can expect to deliver between two and five babies per shift and assist at another four to six births even if they have had no previous training (International School of Midwifery 1997).

Promotional materials for the clinics/trips use the language of tourism to frame the sites as exotic and desirable. Topographies ravaged by the incursions of transnational corporations are rendered whole and unblemished. This is a description of El Paso taken from a clinic brochure: "El Paso is situated in the Chihuahuan desert in the western corner of Texas, on the Texas, New Mexico and Mexico borders. It is very hot and dry in the summer with balmy mild winters; sometimes it even snows. The city is bisected by the Franklin Mountains, which is [sic] at the tail end of the Rocky Mountain chain. This creates a diverse scenery, including spectacular sunrises and sunsets and beautiful mountain views" (Maternidad n.d.). This benign portrait is offered from a border region where the poorest residents on both sides find themselves "breathing the same particulates from open fires, smoke stack emissions, automobile exhausts, burning tires, road dust, and construction sites and sucking water from the same briny depleting aquifers beneath a surface polluted by raw sewage, pesticides and toxic wastes" (Ortega 1991, 2). In a place where both space and identity are subject to frequent and often violent contestation, human interaction is discursively costumed in the garb of contented coexistence: "The term[s] 'bilingual' and 'bicultural' come to life in practically every day-to-day activity in El Paso. With a combined population of over two million, El Paso and its sister city of Cd. Juárez are the largest cities on the US-Mexican border. The constant interaction between the two cities adds up to over a million border crossings per month over the four bridges which connect the US and Mexico" (Maternidad n.d.).

It is more than geography that is reimagined by the narrative strategy used to promote and sustain midwifery tourism. What is most successfully recoded is the positioning of the "tourists" in relation to the "natives." Here, cautious comparisons can be made between midwifery tourism and another form of tourism in which transnational movements and racialized and gendered processes of representation collude – the sex tourism industry in Asia. Care must be exercised in such a comparison. While brutal treatment of Mexican women was witnessed by Canadian midwives in the border clinics, sex tourism exposes the women who are its objects to far more grievous forms of sustained violence, including physical assault, HIV/AIDS infection, and involuntary confinement (Seabrook 1996). What links these two forms of tourism, however, is that in both cases, Third World women's bodies are viewed as a natural resource and "customers lured by an appealing conflation of natural, social and cultural forces are themselves represented as inherently desirable" (Bishop and Robinson 1998, 10).

As Ryan Bishop and Lillian Robinson (1998) have demonstrated in the case of the heterosexual sex trade in Thailand, the conditions of globalization that thrust women into prostitution are thoroughly obscured through Thai women's representation in tourist literature as naturally desirous of sexual commerce with white men, a representation that also serves to explain the low cost and easy availability of these women for paid sexual encounters. The identical discursive dynamic can be viewed in the midwifery tourism pamphlet quoted above. Having rendered neutral the harsh environmental and social realities of the border, having performed a magical disappearance of the entire neocolonial system, promoters of midwifery tourism are able to argue that Mexican mothers freely choose midwifery care in the clinics because it is an "affordable and desirable alternative" (Maternidad n.d.) and not because it is a survival strategy in an environment that offers few options. As in sex tourism discourse, midwifery tourism's key selling points are the availability of abundant desiring and desirable bodies and promises of pleasure for the consumer. A letter accompanying a brochure for potential interns guarantees, in protopornographic language, access to "a lot of beautiful Mexican Mamas" and promises that the intern can "expect to palpate and listen to more bellies than you ever thought possible ... But most of all you can expect to have fun!" (Milligan n.d.).

Although they position themselves as the generous benefactors of women eager and grateful for contact, midwifery tourists, like sex tourists, reap rewards well beyond those gained by those who service them. Western (male) heterosexual sex tourists return to a privileged existence, their white masculinity secured through sex with brown women. Midwifery tourists, on the other hand, come home endowed with an enhanced respectability that allows them to claim a relatively lofty slot in a race- and gender-segmented workforce. Those who enable these rewards, however, merely survive. This unequal exchange is at the heart of transnational logic. "Whether the gift is worth the price for which the receiver has to pay," Trinh T. Minh-ha (1991, 22) has commented, "is a long term question which not every gift giver asks." To do so would unveil the reigning "mystique of reciprocity" (Bishop and Ryan 1998, 126) to reveal that these tourists' innocence is an illusion.

Narrating the Innocent Tourist
The discursive enticements to midwifery tourism promise a fair exchange, an act of benevolence and a moral project, all of which secure the traveller's innocence rather than reveal her collusion with the violent effects of globalization. However, encounters in the border clinics threaten to undo this perception. Innocence is fundamental to midwifery subjecthood in Ontario where it is narrated through the "heroic tale," wherein a dedicated group of

women endured both legal jeopardy and personal sacrifice to create "not just another profession, but a tool to gain community-based woman-defined care" (Van Wagner 1988a, 117). Some of the challenges threatening this one-sided narrative have been recounted, but it is the "forgetting" of those processes that allows the tale to be told and enables midwives to assume a subjecthood that is unassailably moral and unproblematically unitary. As Teresa de Lauretis (1984, 159) has argued, subjectivity is not a "fixed point of departure or arrival from which one then interacts with the world," but is produced instead through our social interactions and our shifting positions within those interactions. If true, it cannot be the case that experience is something that individuals "have." Rather, experience is the grounds upon which our very subjecthood is articulated.

Subjectivities are produced in relationship; however, they require technologies of articulation to render them intelligible and serviceable. Narrative is one such technology. The structuring of narrative imposes a coherency on the unruly strands of a story by discarding those threads that threaten to disturb the desired pattern of the weave. But the sequencing of this weave, as Hayden White (1981) has pointed out, always assumes a moral ordering. How then do midwifery tourists, through the stories they tell about their experiences in the border clinics, reclaim a moral self by reordering the threads of a narrative that includes participation in forms of care that are at best antithetical to an articulated Ontario midwifery philosophy of female benevolence and of multicultural sensitivity and, at worst, unmistakably violent?

A common thread running through the midwives' narratives of their border experiences is the language barrier between themselves and the Spanish-speaking women they attended. In the promotional materials for one border clinic, "a thorough understanding of English" is required for admission but only a basic understanding of Spanish is deemed necessary. This, despite the fact that 85 percent of the clientele are unilingual Spanish speakers (Maternidad n.d.). In a second clinic, Spanish is "recommended but not required" (Casa de Nacimiento n.d.). Much of the communication between Ontario midwives and Spanish-speaking women in the clinics happens through non-verbal forms of communication that, for the tourist, can be yet another exotic attraction "to be felt internally, recognized and enjoyed as a private and intensified 'object'" (Curtis and Pajaczkowska 1994, 207). The Ontario midwives I interviewed were convinced of the authenticity of their interpretations of the communication conducted through non-verbal cues and improper Spanish usage; these communication gaps were most frequently construed as benign. Such a construction resolves the contradiction inherent in Ontario midwives' providing care under inferior communicative conditions even when education and counselling, shared decision making, and informed choice are the hallmarks of midwifery care in the province (College of Midwives of Ontario 1994).

Ineffective communication between Spanish-speaking women and their Anglo-Canadian caregivers as a humorous event is a frequent theme in the interview narratives. "They're amazing people actually," remarked one veteran midwife, referring to the women she cared for. "They're so warm in terms of being accepting, especially of students who speak poor Spanish. They used to laugh at me all the time" (Interview no. 21). Communication barriers were found to be not just amusing, but therapeutic as well. One midwife told me, "I would make a lot of those Mexican ladies laugh their heads off all night long listening to me attempt to speak Spanish. It was really good to help them open up [achieve cervical dilation]. They thought it was really funny" (Interview no. 18). Another found it "hilarious" to be working in an environment that was Spanish-speaking when she spoke only a rudimentary form of the language (Interview no. 24).

Whether care in a border clinic is benevolent and humane (as it frequently is) or tinged by violence (as in the experiences described by some of those interviewed), the relationship between Mexican women and white midwives is always embedded in a transnational and local racial hierarchy. For Mexican women using the border clinics, compliance and laughter might represent a spontaneous display of mirth, but such behaviour might also symbolize an indispensable survival strategy learned in a hostile border space. Cross-cultural communication, argues Ofelia Schutte (1998, 53), is often received in fragments, and it is frequently the most important part of the message that is discarded because its accurate reception would require "the radical decentring of the dominant Anglophone speaking subject." In at least one study of Latina women's childbearing experience in the United States, laughter was not the response the researchers encountered when women relayed the impact of language on their maternity care. Rather, Carolyn Sargent and Grace Bascope (1997, 193) report that during interviews with Spanish-speaking women after childbirth in a Texas hospital, "several women cried upon realizing that the interviewer spoke Spanish, expressing their desperation to find someone with whom they could communicate."

Two of the women interviewed described witnessing events in the border clinics which transformed their experience from a demonstration of their dedication to the profession to a test of their moral and physical resolve to gain midwifery experience. The women were clear about their objections to what they witnessed but still attempted to resolve the contradictions between the unnerving realities of the border internships and their own benevolent self-conceptions. Their strategies range from, in one case illustrated below, constructing a subtle narrative that distinguishes the witnessing student from the guilty perpetrators of the violence, to constructing a blanket rationale in which the repellent elements of the training are justified by the acquisition of valuable midwifery experience.

An Ontario midwife describes her astonishment and disgust at the violent treatment a Mexican woman receives, but quickly elides that violence by recoding herself as a potential victim of the vicious behaviour of the clinic's midwives. In this way, she manages to justify both her self-imposed silence and her continued stay at the clinic:

The hardest part for me was after being there for two weeks, seeing the director kind of say to women [harshly spoken], "Get up on the bed" with her knee like this, like *tooph*, like getting really impatient with this woman [shouting], "Open your legs, *ahh aah ahh!*" And I just thought ... what am I doing here? This is awful! I've got to speak to this. So we're sitting around the table afterwards chewing the fat and I just ... "You know I feel that it's really important ... I don't feel that any woman in labour should ever be treated unkindly." "Oh," says C, "um-hmm." "Oh," says R, the other intern. Silence. Then they decided they were going to blackball me, kick me out of the program. How dare I critique the program? So, very early on, I got my threat, you know. And I never ever opened my mouth about anything that I couldn't stand there. (Interview no. 19)

In another incident, the Ontario midwife quoted above describes the behaviour at a birth of a clinic employee whom she knew to engage in casual prostitution. The speaker emphasizes the clinic midwife's unrespectable status by referencing her as a prostitute and biker and masculinizes her by describing her behaviour in the language of sexual violence and male esprit de corps. As the narrative describes the "prostitute woman," it simultaneously constructs, by contrast, the femininity, innocence, empathic character, and middle-class sensibilities of the speaker, masking her complicity in the violent scene: "You know the 'rape' began and the woman in the Harley-Davidson T-shirt, the prostitute woman in the Harley-Davidson T-shirt, put her feet up against the wall and her knee in the woman's belly to push the baby out and the blood flowed, and her mother-in-law came with her Kleenex to cry and mop up the blood. It was just awful. There was this sort of camaraderie, this sort of rough camaraderie afterwards: 'Oh, did you see her mother-in-law was praying?'; gross stuff, gross stuff" (Interview no. 19).

For many of those interviewed, descriptions of their border experiences are deeply infused with ambivalence. One woman returned with a "real sense of experimenting on people" (Interview no. 36). She was particularly disturbed by the transformation of birthing women's bodies into a spectacle where up to ten people would pile into a labour room to observe the final moments of birth. "Sometimes it's kind of like a 'crotch on a plate,'" she told me. "I mean, you come in there for ten minutes. I mean, what have you seen? Have you seen a birth? No. Have you seen a baby come out? Yes"

(Interview no. 36). Others described being profoundly disturbed by the lack of respect and absence of choice that characterized the care in which they participated. However ambivalent they felt about their stays in the border clinics and in Third World practice sites, all the women considered their experiences to be invaluable. They were described as "good," "great," and "inspirational." Those who had witnessed the most violent incidents were adamant that even if they had known beforehand what it would be like, they would still have gone to the clinics.

The Rewards of Midwifery Tourism

Ontario midwives and students who went to border clinics were unanimous in their recognition of the material and discursive value of the experience. During the early years of the midwifery movement in Ontario, this experience increased midwives' credibility not only among peers and clients but among other medical professionals as well. A recent study of the midwifery movement in Ontario notes that the "rewards and actual leadership status was [sic] given in the early days in the Movement in Ontario to those who had very early begun learning about birth through 'life experience' the traditional way midwives used to learn. Third World experience was especially held in high esteem" (Daviss 1999, 107). One woman who had apprenticed with physicians in the 1970s talked about the importance of her lengthy stay at a border clinic. "The significance was that I was considered by the doctors that I worked with when I came back as someone now who had experience, a lot of experience," she recalled. "And most doctors ... just absolutely assumed that I had my equipment ... (and that) I would catch the baby at birth. So it gave me a certain kind of ability, expertise, understanding. I learned a lot, I thought a lot. I dealt with stuff down there. Postpartum haemorrhage that was unbelievable that I'd never dealt with here" (Interview no. 19).

Access to complicated maternity cases was key in conferring a degree of medical expertise and credibility that would have been impossible to acquire in Ontario, where midwives managed only medically uncomplicated births. In an oddly contradictory way, travelling to the border clinics allowed Ontario midwives to claim both medical and midwifery authenticity through their experience with Third World women, whose birthing capacities are ambivalently marked as both natural and pathological in the descriptions. Border clinic experience even served as a tool for convincing reluctant Canadian physicians of midwives' professional skill. Venturing into what must have been exceedingly hostile territory, pro-midwifery Toronto physician Brian Goldman published a 1988 article on home birth in the *Canadian Medical Association Journal* in which the border clinic experience of the midwife and her exposure to abnormal birth are used as evidence of her competence. More recently, the border clinic experience allowed one aspiring midwife "to see a lot of things that I wouldn't see here because of numbers. I mean I saw a prolapsed cord, I saw babies going, I saw a lot of haemorrhages, this and that" (Interview no. 31). For another, Third World women provide a constantly renewable source of expertise: "And what I find ... I've always done is I go back to developing countries to refresh my skills on doing breeches and twins and some of these complicated cases here" (Interview no. 17).

Midwifery tourism is a particularly transparent example of how First World feminists make use of imperial subject positions in their struggle for localized forms of gender justice and how identity is made in and through space. And while midwifery legislation did not directly compel midwives to travel abroad for experience, the conditions for its implementation made midwifery tourism a necessary strategy for some white women seeking to become registered midwives in the province. The enticements and incentives that make these travels desirable, and the rationalizations that render them benevolent, demonstrate the numerous ways in which white First World subjects, even those with relatively little power in the transnational scheme of things, continue to find racialized others a useful tool in constructing dominant identities. Little, if any reward, however, accrues to the women whose availability as objects of study is predicated on globalizing processes of uneven development. Nor are Third World women recognized outside of the imperial script when they appear in the West, not as reified objects of a primitivist discourse, but as agents in their own rights (Alexander 1998).

4
"Ambassadors of the Profession": The Construction of Respectable Midwifery

Because there are myths and, in fact, fears about midwives in our society, it is very important not to alienate the audience by reinforcing any of the myths by your appearance or the content of your speech ... If you appear to fit right into your audience's stereotype of a "backwoods hippie" or "starry-eyed earth mother" with "yellow socks and Birkenstock sandals" or a "strident angry militant feminist" or "selfish homebirth fanatic," then you have defeated the purpose of being there in the first place ... It is very important at this time in the history of midwifery that we present a very consistent vision of what a midwife is. This is not the time for individual visions of midwifery – although hopefully the time is coming.

 – Vicki Van Wagner, "How to Speak about Midwifery Issues"

In a sense, the power of normalization imposes homogeneity; but it individualizes by making it possible to measure gaps, to determine levels, to fix specialties and to render the differences useful by fitting them one to another. It is easy to understand how the power of the norm functions within a system of formal equality, since within a homogeneity that is the rule, the norm introduces, as a useful imperative, and as a result of measurement, all the shading of individual differences.

 – Michel Foucault, *Discipline and Punish*

Immigrant midwives of colour were not the only women who threatened the creation of a respectable midwifery profession. The midwifery movement harboured its own "others" who, as Vicki Van Wagner demonstrates in the opening epigraph, provoked enough alarm to require a concerted strategy of repudiation. To make rights claims on the state and achieve access to both health care resources and public approval, midwives in Ontario required a significant degree of social and epistemological parity with the professional group that is paradigmatic of respectability, power, and scientific rationality: physicians (Starr 1982). Ultimately, midwives needed to attain an ontological positioning in the public imagination as scientific/rational readers of women's reproductive lives (Murphy-Lawless 1998). Veteran midwives who threatened this positioning by virtue of their immoderate spirituality, femininity, or emotionality found themselves pushed to the margins of the midwifery movement. A new norm – in the form of the neutral, liberal humanist subject – was rapidly occluding the figure of excess that had come to be associated with the revival of midwifery in North America. While unruly veteran practitioners were being contained, the production of rational/respectable midwives was being consolidated in the provincial Midwifery Education Programme (MEP), where subjects were disciplined, identities policed, and norms inscribed.

In *Discipline and Punish*, Michel Foucault traces the development of those disciplinary mechanisms that, in an age of putative equality, introduced "insuperable asymmetries and excluding reciprocities." Such mechanisms, he argues, secured the dominance of the bourgeoisie through non-juridical means. Foucault reasons that, in modern times, exclusion cannot be understood to function through a "massive binary division between one set of people and the other." Rather, he claims, it is achieved through "multiple separations, individualizing distributions, an organization in depth of surveillance and control, and an intensification and a ramification of power." Juxtaposing the figure of the leper with that of the plague victim, Foucault describes two separate, but not unrelated, means of differentiation: the construction of the "pure community" and the production of the "disciplined society" (Foucault 1979, 198, 199).

At the heart of all disciplinary projects resides the "normal" individual who serves as a "standard of valuation" for determining who is to be included and who excluded from a given collectivity. This norm, as John S. Ransom (1997, 52) notes, "acts not in a descriptive sense, but in a prescriptive sense, imposing a good-bad distinction on what was at first only a mean distribution of individuals." Such a distinction is candidly drawn by midwifery activist Vicki Van Wagner in the opening epigraph, wherein Ontario midwifery's (white) figures of ill-repute are summoned up against a norm that is invoked in inverse relation to the clutch of disagreeable figures that she sketches. As Edward Said (1993, 52) has argued, cultural identities are never self-referential constructs but form, rather, "contrapuntal ensembles" with their various "opposites, negatives, oppositions." Country/city, material/spiritual, archaic/modern, rational/irrational, disembodied/embodied, public/private are just a few of the binaries alluded to in Van Wagner's quotation. Arguably, it is the first partner in each pair that is favoured in the moral ordering which constructs the norm lurking behind Van Wagner's admonition. Peeking from the shadows is to be found none other than the liberal humanist subject: abstract, autonomous, independent, unraced, and ungendered. This subjectivity, as Margaret Shildrick (1997, 147) argues, requires "taking on the ontological status of a man," a man, I would add, who is always already racially (un)marked as white. This is a subjecthood not available to all. The valorization of this norm and the bending of midwifery subjects toward it has prevented the midwifery professionalization project from delivering a broader liberatory and democratic vision.

Examined here is the project of disciplining white midwives (and the few racialized "others" deemed worthy of inclusion) so as to produce "ambassadors of the profession" (Bourgeault 1996, 129): neutral and rational/scientific subjects whose whiteness and bourgeois character are uncontaminated by figures of abjection. This chapter traces how the decision to pursue state regulation necessitated a particular kind of midwifery subject, and it maps the cultural battles over the construction of the "new midwife." To whom is the new midwifery subjectivity available, and how has midwifery used the modern appeal of "technical-rational rule" (Flax 1993, 42) to exclude its "others"?

Race and the Elimination of the Midwife:
Historical Discontinuities between the United States and Canada

The images that represent midwifery as an archaic and disreputable profession have enjoyed a remarkable longevity. And while opponents of midwifery in both Canada and the United States drew liberally on such negative representations in both recent and past campaigns to impede the practice, they diverged in relationship to their employment of unmistakably racist discourses. Racism was central to the elimination of the midwife in the United States early in the last century, but it has not constituted a significant rhetorical or political strategy in Canadian antimidwifery discourse. Rather, in their evocation of the dangerous midwife, opponents of self-regulating midwifery in Canada employed discourses that conflated the obsolete and the feminine. Consequently, a political strategy that sought to contain those midwives who represented female excess became important to midwifery activists in the struggle for legalization.

The evolving public image of the midwife in the West can be understood as a palimpsest on which has been inscribed a progression of ominous figures, including the witch/midwife portrayed in the infamous *Malleus Maleficarum*, a fifteenth-century text that codified the Catholic Church's anxieties over the links between midwifery and sorcery; Sairey Gamp, the dirty crone of Charles Dickens' 1884 novel *Martin Chuzzlewit*; the "ignorant" granny-midwife who, until the 1960s, continued to deliver many African-American women in the Southern US; the alternately reviled and revered Third World midwife; and finally, the "starry-eyed" hippie midwife. Feminist scholars have, in recent years, launched historiographic challenges to these negative discourses, offering richly complex analyses of midwifery's decline.[1] Popular writers as well have attempted to reconstruct the midwife as a transhistorical/global female folk hero.[2] Such efforts, however, have not entirely succeeded in overturning this archive of disparaging representations. Although a thorough examination of the historically and geographically specific processes that have produced these images is beyond the scope of this chapter, it can be argued that the demise of the traditional midwife in the West and her replacement with the physician, or the physician-supervised nurse-midwife, is coterminous with the decline in traditional anthropomorphic epistemologies and the ascendancy of science in Europe (Papps and Olssen 1997). Such a development must be understood not as an abrupt shift from "superstition and magic to objective scientific knowledge," but seen rather, as Lois McNay (1994, 5) argues, as a "series of abrupt and arbitrary paradigm breaks." Dotted with innumerable pockets of resistance, the overall effect of such breaks was that women and non-European "others" were deemed atavistic repositories of outmoded knowledge while white European men were seen as the "bearers of modernity" (Papps and Olssen 1997, 52).

In the US context, an escalation of antimidwifery sentiment can be traced to the turn of the last century when medical education became standardized and a burgeoning belief in the efficacy of scientific medicine was taking hold among white, middle-class Americans (Arney 1982). Both non-specialist physicians and members of the growing obstetric profession in the United States viewed midwifery as an impediment to their professional, economic, and political advancement. Having already become the *accoucheur* of choice for nearly all white middle-class women in America, the physician still faced competition from immigrant and native-born midwives who continued to deliver the babies of many immigrant and poor urban and rural women (Wertz and Wertz 1989). Nearly 86 percent of Italian-American births were reported by midwives in 1908 (Litoff 1978, 27), and a 1924 study revealed that 86 percent of Minnesota midwives were foreign-born and that they served communities where the majority of residents were immigrants (Borst 1995, 44). And while by 1935 the percentage of women attended by midwives had dropped to 12.5 percent from 50 percent in 1900, nearly 80 percent of those midwives who continued to practise were African-American traditional midwives working in the rural southern United States (Rooks 1997, 30) who would, for a variety of reasons, not be completely eliminated until the 1960s.[3] Unfounded suspicions that midwives contributed to increasing maternal and infant mortality rates were also deeply intertwined, in both Canada and the United States, with the concern with "race degeneration" that arose in response to the influx of immigrants and the high casualty rates of the Second World War.[4] It is not surprising then, that antimidwifery discourse in the United States during the early twentieth century relied heavily on racist and xenophobic themes to discredit the midwife.

However, US antimidwifery discourse of the early twentieth century was superimposed upon an amalgam of older discourses in which the degenerate female figure of Sairey Gamp, the unkempt, unruly, and inebriated proletarian nurse in *Martin Chuzzlewit* figured prominently. Some physician monographs of the time targeted "the typical old, gin-fingering, guzzling midwife with her pockets full of forcing drops, her mouth full of snuff, her fingers foul of dirt and her brains full of arrogance and superstition" (Sullivan and Weitz 1988, 11). However, like Joseph B. DeLee, the most prominent obstetrician of his day and an activist in the movement to eliminate midwives, some physicians employed particularly misogynist forms of racism and xenophobia in their rhetoric. A popular article written by DeLee in 1926 featured depictions and disparaging descriptions of three midwives: an Italian woman, a Southern black woman, and an Irish woman, all dressed in dark garb and portrayed against an ominously dim background. It carried the following descriptions: "A typical Italian midwife practicing in one of our cities. They bring with them filthy customs and practices ... [A] granny of the far South. Ignorant and superstitious, a survival of the magic doctors of the West Coast of Africa ... Surely it might have been this woman of Irish-American parentage who is quoted as having said: 'I am too old to clean, too weak to wash, too blind to sew; but, thank God, I can still put my neighbors to bed'" (Susie 1988, 5).

Such images have enjoyed an extraordinary longevity. Well after midwifery had been virtually eliminated in the United States and Canada, the figure of the degenerate midwife continued to be used by journalists and physicians to trumpet the triumph of obstetrics over the risks of childbirth, and the victory of science over superstition in the lying-in chamber. As late as 1960, the *Ladies' Home Journal* castigated the "unsanitary crone" and celebrated the "long medical struggle against the horrors of much old-fashioned midwifery" (quoted in Miller 1997, 71).

The shadow of race falls differently on the Canadian and American histories of the elimination of the midwife in the nineteenth and twentieth centuries. The campaign to eliminate the midwife in the United States was conspicuously organized around the figures of the immigrant and black-granny midwife at the turn of the century. In Canada, racialized minority women who practised midwifery were left largely unmolested by the state until well into the twentieth century. Aboriginal midwifery is a case in point. Medical missionaries made early incursions aimed at dismantling Aboriginal childbearing systems, but it was only in the 1940s and 1950s that the Medical Services Branch of Health and Welfare Canada instituted coercive tactics forcing Aboriginal people to abandon indigenous health practices such as traditional midwifery (Thomas 1993).[5] There is also evidence that Chinese-Canadian women relied on Chinese midwives and Japanese-Canadian women relied on Japanese-trained community midwives until at least the 1930s and possibly beyond.[6] The role of midwives during the internment of Japanese Canadians during the Second World War is yet to be examined.[7] Such evidence is tantalizingly scant and in need of exploration.

The demise of the midwife in Canada can be loosely understood as the purging of female expertise in childbirth and its replacement by a scientific model of childbirth management (which included important technological innovations such as anaesthesia, Caesarean section, and aseptic technique) propounded by and practised almost exclusively by men. Much historical literature focuses on this process in relation to Ontario, where by the middle of the last century the institution of "social childbirth," in which female relatives, friends, neighbours, and a community midwife attended the labouring woman, had been replaced by hospital-based childbirth managed by physicians (Mason 1987; Biggs 1990; Oppenheimer 1990).[8] As in the United States, the elimination of the midwife came on the heels of the consolidation of medical "regulars" and the enactment of legislation that prevented unlicensed practitioners from performing medical acts (Biggs 1990). There is a debate among Canadian historians as to whether the disappearance of midwifery is attributable primarily to physician opposition and a concerted campaign of eradication, or whether demographic, geographic, and technological factors played an equally or more important role in midwifery's demise. What is certain, however, is that midwives largely ceased to practise by early in the last century.[9] In Ontario, for example, by 1897 the overwhelming majority of births were managed by physicians, and by 1938 most women were giving birth in hospitals (Oppenheimer 1990, 56).

Early in the last century, the National Council of Women initiated a scheme to address the lack of trained childbirth assistants for rural women that aroused strident opposition to the profession (Buckley 1979; Boutilier 1994). The scheme intended to provide midwifery training to local women, augmented by instruction in "first aid, simple nursing and 'household economy and sanitation'" (Mason 1987, 210). Both physicians and trained nurses expressed intractable resistance to the scheme. Just as physicians did not wish to endanger their professional dominance over birth, newly professionalized nurses, having put to rest the Sairey Gamp legacy, were equally unwilling for nursing labour to be associated in any way with domestic work. Both physicians and nurses employed rhetoric that linked midwives with "dirt, ignorance and danger" in their efforts to prevent the training or importation of midwives (Boutilier 1994, 34). United in their opposition and mindful of whom they wished to build the nation, physicians and nurses feared that schemes to import British midwives would allow "old country people who know nothing of our conditions to dictate a solution of our problems by dumping on to our prairies people they wish to get rid of" (Mary Ard MacKenzie [1917] quoted in Buckley 1979, 143). Opponents of midwifery registered a figure of abjection that was hopelessly female, proletarian, and old-world and was mired in an atavistic form of domestic empirical knowledge far removed from science's promise to deliver women from the perils and indignities of childbirth. In the late nineteenth and early twentieth centuries, she was precisely the figure against whom professional nurses marked their respectability and physicians their scientific rationality and consequent entitlement to manage the bodies of women.

Even though Canadian physicians were largely unconcerned with midwifery for much of the twentieth century, negative images still surfaced and began, in the 1970s, to appear with increasing frequency. In 1970, at the very moment that the counterculture/feminist midwifery revival was making its debut, a book review published in the *Canadian Medical Association Journal* (*CMAJ*) claimed that "the term [midwife] has a stigma attached to it. It conjures up a picture of an old, unhygienic, unscientific granny, delivering babies in the backwoods, relying heavily on superstition and magic elixirs" (Bruser 1970, 762). As Winkup (1998, 70) has shown in her review of *CMAJ* articles relating to midwifery that appeared between 1967 and 1997, much rhetoric by Canadian physicians deemed midwifery to be "medically obsolescent" and they frequently voiced opposition to home birth. Ontario physicians were also opposed to home birth but not to the legalization of midwives. Their stance diverged from that of the Canadian Medical Association, which published its official position opposing the licensing of midwives in 1987, a year after the Ontario Ministry of Health announced its intention to regulate midwives and the year that the landmark *Report of the Task Force on the Implementation of Midwifery in Ontario* was published. Responses to the Association's position in the pages of the *CMAJ* frequently evoked midwifery as an outdated practice. For those seeking to discredit midwives, the confluences between older negative representations of midwifery and the emergent "counterculture" empirical midwives could be logically posited. These confluences were to prove problematic for the midwifery movement. Those midwives who viewed the forgotten "neighbour-midwife" not as a skeleton in midwifery's closet but as an ideal to be emulated, and for whom midwifery practice was part of the achievement of a holistic pastoral ideal and not a professionalization project, would find themselves struggling for credibility, respect and, ultimately, the right to continue to practise.

New Midwifery Identities, Old Midwifery Images

Beginning in the 1970s a vigorous counternarrative to the obstetrical saga of maternal safety and satisfaction began to arise in the United States, Canada, and Great Britain.[10] Empirical midwifery and home birth, virtually eliminated in the first half of the century, were enjoying a revival among some North American white women. British midwives, who had not been eliminated in the twentieth century but had come under medical regulation, began to challenge the increasing medicalization of their profession with the establishment in 1976 of the Association for Radical Midwives (Weitz 1987), and US nurse-midwifery, which had somehow managed to survive the century, saw a doubling of its clientele (Rooks 1997).[11] Part of an overall undermining of medical authority, the anti-obstetrical movements had their own unique trajectory. The popular childbirth reform movement reflected a curious convergence of ideologies ranging from the cultural Left's critiques of the fragmentation of modern life and its separation from nature, to the feminist health movement's advocacy of medical self-help and women's right to reproductive choice, to the gender traditionalism and heteronormativity of breastfeeding advocates like the La Leche League, to religious fundamentalists' refusal of state intervention into the childbearing process. All of these elements are in evidence in the Ontario midwifery movement, where "counterculture" midwives and supporters exerted a powerful influence in the years before legislation. However, this vision of midwifery was not to survive the political struggles of the ensuing decade. Those who sought to preserve "unregulated organic midwifery ... which is grounded on spiritual and humanitarian premises and grows naturally from group conscience" (Monk 1995, 7) – the "backwoods hippies," "starry-eyed earth mothers," and "strident home birth fanatics" – found themselves embattled within a movement whose claims to legitimacy were increasingly grounded not only in the authoritative discourses of science, but in claims to a general social normativity.

"Counterculture" Influences in the Re-emergence of Midwifery

In one of several prelegislation monographs in which she argued that state regulation was wholly antithetical to the spirit of community-based midwifery in Ontario,[12] historian and midwifery supporter Jutta Mason (1989, 5) described seeing photographs of midwife Judi Pustil delivering her first child in 1979: "The pictures were taken in a summer meadow beside a stream near Powassan; about a half a dozen friends stood or sat in the grass beside Judi. One of them held an open book. Judi told us – amid much laughter – that they were all so 'green' concerning birth that when the baby's head started to show, all wrinkled, everyone thought it was a bum and they hastily looked up the section on breech birth." Stories like this arose frequently in the interviews that I conducted with veteran white midwives. Although this sort of narrative has been supplanted by the "heroic tale" of midwifery, it serves for some as the mythological origin story of midwifery in Ontario. Constrained neither by doctors and patriarchal medicine, as in the hospital, *nor* by the expertise of empirically trained and occasionally medically trained home-birth midwives, Pustil's outdoor birth is presided over by none other than Mother Nature herself. This birth and those of other women attended by "untrained workers," argued Mason (1989, 6), contributed to the growing store of "exemplary birth statistics" not only achieved through the efforts of lay midwives, but attributable as well to the counterculture approach to pregnancy, birth, and child care. A clear refutation of the claims of obstetrical and other medical practitioners that medicalization had reduced the risks of childbirth, these statistics, she said, reflected not luck, but "the genius of the alternative birth culture: the joy, the neighbourly connections we revived, the crazy quilt of diets, chants, politics, sleeping-in-one bed: all of it, not one element, not even mainly midwives." Even Vicki Van Wagner, who was to be instrumental in the implementation of both midwifery legislation and university-based education for midwives, still clung, in 1982, to the belief that professional expertise was not at the heart of community midwifery in Ontario. "Part of our struggle," explained Van Wagner, "has been to recognize that our support as women and mothers, not particularly as experts, can help women in pregnancy and labour" (Van Wagner quoted in Mason 1989, 3).

While Ontario childbirth reformers did reflect the divergent ideologies apparent in the rest of the North American movement, much promidwifery literature in the years prior to the province's decision in 1985 to legalize midwifery echoed Mason's "countercultural" views. The pages of *Re-Birth*, a "quarterly newspaper about choices in childbirth," published by midwifery supporters for several years in the mid-1980s, were filled, for example, with ads for natural foods stores and cloth diapers, as well as with critical reviews of the medical policies of the province's hospitals, "miraculous" home-birth stories, suggestions for herbal remedies, and directions for "natural family planning." The antimedical stance of much of the paper's editorial copy is unmistakable.

Among the many cross-border influences was the extraordinary success of Ina May Gaskin's 1975 book, *Spiritual Midwifery*. Gaskin, an empirically trained midwife from Tennessee, wrote about birth on The Farm, a rural commune in Summertown, Tennessee, that she had founded in 1971 with her husband, Stephen, and several hundred followers who joined them in pursuit of the "hippie pastorale – a life of minimal technology ... self-determination and the happy coexistence of human life with nature" (Umansky 1996, 54). A combination of how-to guide for midwives and an anthology of personal narratives emphasizing the spiritual elements of the childbirth experience, the book sold over half a million copies in the United

States and Canada over twenty years (Rooks 1997, 61). A stunning advocacy of the evident safety of home birth for healthy, well-nourished women,[13] the book also accomplished a unique, perhaps unprecedented, recuperation of the language of birth from medical experts. Uterine contractions in labour were neologized as "rushes" and recast as exhilarating and sensual rather than painful and frightening. The euphoric language of the psychedelic drug culture and clear references to sexual behaviour also figured prominently in the book's "amazing birth tales": "Well, I got behind Judith and leaned her head on my chest and kind of cradled her and rubbed and kissed her and did stuff to turn her on again ... And shortly she was rushing all kinds of pretty rushes and color changes. She changed colors in waves usually starting in heavy pink at her head and moving down in about an eight-inch wide wave followed by a gold and a white, the pink one being very physically visible and the other being more like shining light around her" (Gaskin 1978,193). In touch with midwives in Ontario, Gaskin saw the holistic birth culture as imperilled by the move to legislation. Addressing followers in Toronto in 1989, she warned that professionalization would "cut off opportunities to learn from every unique woman" and block access to "women's collective knowledge" (Monk 1994, 9).

Gaskin's book introduced counterculture midwifery and the figure of the "hippie" midwife to hundreds of thousands of readers. And while *Spiritual Midwifery* is not an overtly antimedical text, it powerfully reclaims and renames obstetrical knowledge, peels away its scientific skin, and harnesses it firmly to non-rationalist thought and feminine essentialism.[14] Those who wished to could easily have argued that the continuities between the hippie midwife and her disreputable predecessors were practically seamless. So close was the confluence, that in her tribute to the virtues of Canada's emerging midwives, *Midwifery Is Catching*, Eleanor Barrington (1985, 16) felt compelled to account for Gaskin's "spiritual midwife." "A source of much honest confusion," wrote Barrington, "the spiritual midwife works with birth as part of the ebb and flow of life, acknowledging the forces beyond the physical process. But she is not a witch doctor who merely voices incantations when action is required." Untrained, superstitious, and even racialized in Barrington's reference to the witch doctor, the hippie midwife constituted another inscription upon the midwifery palimpsest and yet another disagreeable subjectivity against which midwifery respectability in Ontario would have to be crafted.

In the years just prior to the province's decision to legalize midwifery, midwives were treated to a timely reminder that older antimidwifery discourses had not been abandoned, that women's projects that sought to defy the authority of scientific medicine would not go unchallenged, and that midwives' apparent epistemological marginality left them vulnerable to public attack. In *A History of Women's Bodies*,[15] Canadian historian Edward

Shorter (1982, 35) launched a powerful salvo against *"engagé* scholars in the women's movement who see the midwives of the past as a great boon to womankind." Shorter's openly stated and immensely curious intent in the book is to demonstrate that contrary to feminist critiques, modern medicine actually enabled the emergence of feminism by improving women's health. "Traditional women's culture," claims Shorter, did not represent a pre-modern utopia, but was actually the source of much of women's suffering. The elimination of that culture's emblematic figure, the midwife, he argues, has been in women's best interest. Only in partnership with men, says Shorter, has women's progress taken place. He devotes an entire chapter of the book to displaying evidence that "golden age" historiography of midwifery is a deception and that, from the sixteenth century onward, "unfavorable opinions about the midwives [came] from all over Europe and Britain until virtually the beginning of the twentieth century." Shorter's accounts of midwifery incompetence are brimming with gruesome detail. "Many traditional midwives," he recounts (1982, 87), "seemed to have been conversant with the knives, sharp hooks (crochets) and blunt hooks needed to decapitate the infant or evacuate its cranium." Shorter (1991, 98) claims elsewhere that if midwives attended most births in the past, and it is known that many women died in childbirth, then midwives must have been responsible for their deaths. This, he suggests, is "the most stunning of any indictment of the traditional midwives."

Published in the same year as a high-profile coroner's inquest into a midwife-attended home birth in the Kitchener-Waterloo area in which a baby subsequently died, *A History of Women's Bodies* appeared at a critical time in the re-emergence of midwifery in Canada. Shorter's intervention into the debate over the practice is not a frivolous one. Methodologically flawed but well researched, *A History of Women's Bodies* draws on a vast and obscure cache of historical literature in several languages. Widely reviewed in both the popular and the academic press, the book seemed to prove, as the *New York Times* reviewer noted, that the "benevolent midwife" was largely mythological (Papps and Olssen, 57). Its impact did not go unnoticed among midwifery supporters in Ontario, who saw the book's publication as a direct threat to the struggle for legitimization. Judging from her references to *A History of Women's Bodies* in an article entitled "Survival tactics for midwives," published in the Spring 1983 edition of *Issue* (the newsletter of the Ontario Association of Midwives), Louise Norman[16] regarded Shorter's work as a direct hit: "Edward Shorter and his much publicized new book pompously reaffirms [sic] the status quo. In print he gets away with 'nobody dies anymore' and on the air 'modern feminists want to go back to having their babies in huts.' Well we know such statements are hogwash, but again thousands will believe him because he's a scholar and because they have never heard or read anything to the contrary. *In the end, public sentiment is the crucial issue*" (Norman 1983, 7, emphasis in the original). Norman correctly locates Shorter's work within a discernible power/knowledge nexus, admitting that the image of midwives as "dirty and primitive" had not been expunged from the public record and that those with little access to public discourse would be hard pressed to create a counternarrative as powerful as the one that Shorter offers. If midwives and their supporters needed a warning that female irrationality would not be tolerated as the basis of a self-regulating, state-funded health care profession, Shorter had provided a highly amplified one.

Disciplining Unruly Midwives in the Pre-integration Period

By the mid-1980s the dominant impulse among members of the Association of Ontario Midwives, their supporters, and many legislators was toward state regulation of midwifery and its integration into the health care system. As Beth Rushing (1993) has argued, Canadian midwifery worked to establish itself in the health care system by propounding both science *and* feminism as its key ideological constructs. A standardized midwifery curriculum, delivered at the university level with "an emphasis on immediate and ongoing clinical experience under supervision" was supported by the Association of Ontario Midwives in its third submission to the Health Professions Legislation Review in 1985 (Bourgeault 1996, 132). As Ivy Bourgeault has pointed out, these changes were not externally imposed but rather voluntarily embraced by the activist midwives who used their political acumen to re-script Ontario midwifery so as to make it acceptable to both the state and the other health care professions upon whose approval midwifery integration hinged. Tolerance for ideological diversity within midwifery was eroding, and in 1985 it began to wear thin, as another coroner's inquest, this time into the death of an infant at a midwife-attended home birth on Toronto Island, made news headlines, bringing midwives under unprecedented public scrutiny. Forced to defend itself on medicine's home turf, the midwifery community employed medical rhetoric and used medical experts in this very public, and ultimately successful, struggle to prove its legitimacy. "Throughout the process," explains Bourgeault (1996, 70), "midwives felt the need to stress their educational background, to dress a certain way to enhance their appearance as professionals, and not to appear to be the 'lunatic fringe' they were originally considered to be."

Midwives' reliance on the ideologies of science and feminism and their disciplining of appearance and demeanour to "professional" norms raises pressing questions about the effects of the liberal state's granting of increased power to women. "Do these expanding relationships," queries Wendy Brown, "produce only active political subjects or do they also produce regulated, subordinated and disciplined state subjects?" As Brown argues, those who are recognized and granted rights by the state require the "stuff of liberal personhood – legal, economic or civil personality." The midwifery activists' embrace of scientific rationality, bourgeois educational norms, and normative female appearance helped secure access to the liberal personhood that rights claims require. Such a strategy provides evidence that, as Brown fears, gains for women granted by the liberal state have a disciplinary effect, producing some subjects who may be political and active but who are also disciplined into certain modes of political agency and subjectivity. If, in order for women to be constituted as liberal subjects, they must "repudiate or transcend the social construction of femaleness" and "enter civil society on socially male terms," then those who viewed midwifery neither as primarily a political crusade nor a public profession, but as an extension of their spirituality and of their legitimate social roles as wives, mothers, friends, neighbours, and so on represented something of a political liability (Brown 1995, 172, 182, 183). If midwives needed to represent the embodiment of liberal subjectivity in order to be seen as legitimate political agents, then those midwives who fell short of that norm needed either to be bent toward it, or else purged. Such was the process applied to practising midwives before and during the grandparenting-in process.

Rural Midwives of Eastern Ontario
More than 120 midwives applied to the Michener Institute Pre-registration Program set up to grandparent-in practising midwives in the months prior to legalization. This number was much higher than the figure of seventy-five estimated by the curriculum development committee in its 1990 report. Seventy-two applicants were ultimately admitted to the program and sixty-three graduated in the fall of 1993. Some of the nine midwives who were left behind felt that they had received biased treatment at the hands of the foreign midwife-assessors (Bourgeault 1996). Among those not admitted to the Michener program were approximately sixteen women, including nine community midwives and seven birthing centre nurses, who organized themselves into the Committee for More Midwives. They vigorously lobbied the provincial government and the midwifery bureaucracy for special consideration of their skills and community responsibilities and for the creation of a special route of entry to the profession. Such consideration was not granted, and for those left out of the Michener program, there remained only two options: to apply for entry to the baccalaureate-granting Midwifery Education Program or wait for the establishment of the Prior Learning Assessment program, where their previous experience could be assessed. The Committee for More Midwives raised troubling questions about how midwifery was being implemented in the province and about who was constituted as a suitable "ambassador of the profession."

In addition to my own critique of the race politics of the preregistration program, other researchers have raised questions about the process by which candidates were chosen for the Michener Institute's program, suggesting that criteria were applied unevenly to program applicants (Monk 1994; Bourgeault 1996; Daviss 1999). One excluded midwife wrote of the transitional period, "Those midwives expressing dissent with the dominant discourse are 'hounded' up front. During the transition to regulated midwifery, they are being refused access to impartial assessment and/or registration despite demonstrated professional competence and extremely supportive client communities" (Monk 1994, 17).

At the very least, the process left some apparently competent midwives unable to practise and some areas of the province with no access to midwifery care. Some of the nurse-midwives who had worked in the province's experimental hospital birth centres failed to gain access because of lack of home-birth and primary care experience; the selection process also seemed to cull a large percentage of women from Eastern Ontario, admitting only three out of the fourteen of the midwives who had been practising in that region, and none of those from rural districts where midwifery was popular. Although Toronto and national media trumpeted the triumph of midwifery legislation in January of 1994, news media in Ottawa and Eastern Ontario were far more circumspect. The *Ottawa Citizen* of 3 January 1994 carried a headline that read "Eastern Ontario faces shortage of midwives," while the *Ottawa Sun* on the same date proclaimed "Out of a job ... angry midwives thrown out of work by new provincial regulations say the rules are flawed and will today demand a review." In rural Eastern Ontario, the reception for legalized midwifery was even chillier. The *Smiths Falls Record News* of 12 January 1994 carried the headline "Rejection of midwives in Lanark County is a lost labour of love" (quoted in Daviss 1999, 207).

Eastern Ontario midwives and their supporters had posed a threat to midwifery respectability for some time. The October 1986 hearings of the Task Force on the Implementation of Midwifery in Ontario (TFIMO), which took place in Kingston, were, according to one midwife, "regarded as one of the places where people 'let their hair down,' where midwives and parents said what they really thought instead of what they were supposed to say to appear 'manageable to the Task Force people.'" Their unorthodox views did not go unnoticed by task force members, who apparently voiced concerns to those midwives who had key roles in the legislative process. One Eastern Ontario midwife recalled being later reprimanded by a board member of the Association of Ontario Midwives after TFIMO chair Allan Schwartz reportedly pronounced that "those midwives up there will never be legalized" (Daviss 1999, 170).

Parts of Eastern Ontario had long been home to those who sought alternative and/or communal lifestyles in which self-sufficiency, including a reliance on community midwives, was valued. In an undated press release, which announced a 3 January 1994 press conference to protest the exclusion of rural Eastern Ontario midwives from practice in the wake of the passage of the Midwifery Act, members of the Lanark Midwifery Support Association protested that the state was extending its reach coercively into their lives. They argued that their preference for midwifery care and their decision to live in rural Ontario were part of their quest for personal freedom. "Once again," they alleged, "legislation from an unmandated bureaucracy is interfering, removing our freedom of choice and NOT serving the people." Their midwives, they claimed, had impeccable safety records and high client satisfaction rates. The plight of the region's midwives was supported by local physicians who had written dozens of letters protesting their exclusion from the registration process (Daviss 1999). Invoking historical forms of midwifery persecution, Lanark County midwifery supporters accused the midwifery establishment of engaging in a "witch hunt." The "backwoods hippie" and "starry-eyed earth mother" appeared to be facing the same fate as her spiritual forebears.[17] Although some were never summarily excluded and others succeeded eventually in becoming registered, those midwives whose inclinations and ideologies resembled those of the Lanark County midwifery supporters faced a less than welcoming environment as midwifery built a state-funded and regulated apparatus in the province.

Non-elite White Midwives in the Legalization Struggle

Eight white midwives who considered themselves socially, politically, or ideologically estranged from midwifery's political elite were interviewed for this project. More the "starry-eyed earth mother," "backwoods hippie," or "selfish home-birth fanatic" than "strident angry militant feminist," these women, many of whom had played key roles in reviving midwifery practice, identified a range of beliefs and behaviours for which they felt marginalized once the midwifery community acceded to the push for professionalization exerted by some of its members. Of the eight, five were legally practising at the time of the interview. Two of these midwives had not succeed in being accepted to the Michener Institute Pre-registration Program, but had entered midwifery through the Prior Learning Assessment/ Prior Learning and Experience Assessment or through the Midwifery Education Program. Of the three midwives interviewed who ultimately completed the Michener program, two who had active practices for many years and met all of the criteria for admission reported being scrutinized overzealously in the grandparenting-in process. For one of these women, whose entry to practice was delayed, "it was like going into mourning! I was in a total panic for about two years trying to figure out what had happened and realizing how far my colleagues had gone to get rid of me"

(Interview no. 17). Of the three trained but non-practising midwives interviewed, one tried several times to enter the profession through the Midwifery Education Program but was denied admission each time. The remaining two midwives chose not to pursue registration.

While my purpose in interviewing this group was to find a theory for their repudiation by the midwifery elite, on several occasions I was treated to a demonstration of one of the key theoretical assertions of this project: that those who are themselves marginalized frequently cling to their own marginalization as a way of refusing implication in systems of domination. Some midwives interviewed, particularly those who had faced barriers to registration, continued to harbour deep resentment toward midwifery's elite. One interviewee referred to the group at the centre of the midwifery implementation bureaucracy in unmistakably masculinist terms, calling them the "gang" and "crew"; another referred to the elites as "femi-nazis." These women were eager to talk to me, I felt, because I was engaged in a project that criticized this group. This dynamic yielded franker data than what might have been collected by a researcher engaged in a less explicitly critical project. However, I was frequently struck (and often made to feel disingenuous) by these women's enthusiasm for my project, which they understood to be an indictment of the elite midwives and vindication of the "good" excluded white midwives whom the elite had wronged. Only a few of those interviewed were willing to see *both* their subordinate positioning as unruly "others" *and* their dominant positioning as white women.

When relating their stories of exclusion, some midwives expressed exclusionary/racist sentiments toward immigrant midwives of colour. One woman described to me her reluctance to employ a second midwife of colour in her practice even though the midwife of colour she currently employed was working only casually as a second attendant and not as a registered midwife:

> I just got a call from a woman of a certain ethnospecific background who wants to join our practice ... but one of my reticences in letting her come and join the practice is that there's already a second attendant in our community who is fulfilling the role of a second attendant at these births. [There's no room for] both of them, specifically with this ethnospecific group, no! 'Cause there aren't enough births coming from it ... I could take her on anyway and have her doing births with everybody ... that's the obvious. But I'm just not sure, we ... already have a practice that's pretty diversified. (Interview no. 17)

This sense of being besieged by "too many" women of colour, together with the belief that women of colour are best suited to practising in their "own communities" were freely articulated. This midwife saw no problem in expressing these attitudes to another white woman, despite having signed the requisite release form in which the antiracist intentions of the research were explicitly stated. Alice McIntyre (1997) argues that such "white talk" is based on an assumption of shared racist attitudes among white people and is, not infrequently, a feature of their conversations. Encounters with openly racist expression, as I can testify, are problematic for the white antiracist researcher. To leave racist expressions unchallenged is to legitimate them, which I most certainly did when I refrained from responding to the midwife's comments. To disagree openly, or to end an interview in which racism is expressed, on the other hand, might restrict the collection of data that provide the basis for a broader analysis of racist processes (Wetherell and Potter 1992). When such issues arose during the interviews, they served as timely reminders that subordinate/dominant are always relational positionings in the social matrix, and as such they need to be historicized.

Motherhood and Midwives
The non-elite white midwives I interviewed identified several features of their own identities they felt set them apart from the elite. The commitment of many women to a style of mothering that prescribed close physical and emotional contact (including prolonged breastfeeding) with infants and young children created a discomfort with the disruptions to family life required by the model of twenty-four-hour on-call midwifery practice to which many midwives subscribed. Some also felt that their mainstream or New Age spiritual beliefs caused them to be marginalized by elite midwives who had demonstrated a sort of hyperrationalism in their quest for legitimization. Finally, a preference for the modes of dress of the North American hippie subculture of the 1960s and 1970s was often mentioned as a point of contention between the elite midwives and those who felt excluded from the political centre. The visual dimension of respectability seems to have played a rather over-determined role in the re-emergence of midwifery and its significance should not be minimized.

Maternal obligations and the espousal of a traditional model of mothering set some of those interviewed apart from many midwifery leaders who emerged in the prelegislation period. Many of these non-elite women were also older than the emergent leadership and, unlike them, had several children and numerous domestic responsibilities that made participating in both midwifery politics *and* midwifery practice nearly impossible (Bourgeault 1996, 46). For some women, the practice of midwifery alone presented difficult ideological and logistical challenges inasmuch as midwives who believed fervently in full-time motherhood frequently needed to leave their children with friends, relatives, or other caretakers. One woman described her ambivalence toward the prelegislation trend toward professionalization: "I was still a mother who was at home with her kids and [...] I didn't want to be this professional that put her kids in day care and that this was more important to her than being with her kids! [...] It's not like I never shuffled my kids off; I did. But I also took them around a lot and, you know, I had my daughter at births when she was a baby and that was one of the biggest and most difficult struggles of being a midwife was also being a mother who was involved" (Interview no. 20). Another woman who had medical midwifery training and who contemplated but decided against practising in Ontario in the early 1980s felt that she was judged deficient because she held normative views of the family:

> I remember going to ... AOM meetings and at one point a midwife ... who I had a very friendly relationship with asked me about whether I was going to have children or not and I sort of said, "Well, I'd like to have a partner first." And [she said], "Are you one of those women who has to have a partner to have children?" YES! ... That was obviously considered like ... I was less of a woman, I guess. I don't know. That I was somehow deficient. That I needed to be supported ... I just think that for me, when I chose to parent, I chose to parent ... I wanted to be available for my kids. (Interview no. 22)

Another midwife was harshly critical of the Ontario model of midwifery as unfriendly to families, which she consciously defines, in the quote below, both inside and outside of heterosexual parameters:

> I heard [a midwifery leader] say ... "If you're a midwife, it's the absolute centre of your life, nothing comes before it. That's what makes a real midwife" ... But for some of us, our families come first ... And I'm sure that for a lot of lesbian relationships, especially if they have children, their families come first! ... I have no choice. I must practise full time. I must practise it to the corporate culture image. Work to the exclusion of all else. Because this is what creates a "real professional," somebody who is willing to sacrifice their family, their fun, their physical health, and their mental stability for their corporate performance! These people are adopting models that are being abandoned left, right, and centre by pretty well every other field. (Interview no. 18)

The centring of professional rather than maternal identity, was, as this midwife recognizes, a key strategy in the legalization of midwifery. Those women whose lives and outlooks were defined more by domestic interdependency than by civil autonomy constituted questionable liberal subjects and feeble claimants to state resources. Wendy Brown (1995, 183) reminds us that in order to be constituted as liberal subjects, women must "abstract from their daily lives in the household and repudiate or transcend the social construction of femaleness consequent to this dailiness." Ambivalent or unruly midwives who wished to continue practising midwifery after legislation found themselves bent, sometimes against their explicit desire, toward this norm of liberal subjecthood. In a cogent example of how disciplinary regimes work at the micro level, midwife Mary Sharpe described, in a 1993 monograph, her midwifery practice group, which had "pioneered the renaissance of midwifery care in Ontario." Composed largely of former teachers who had "many children, had homebirths and breastfed our children until beyond toddlerhood," the group, in the wake of legislation, had to "get ourselves organized. We understand now that expertise in academia and politics as well as experience and midwifery skill is important in order to 'move ahead' in the current midwifery community. What previously was a matter of philosophical preference is now a matter of power around real decisions that affect our lives" (Sharpe 1993, 10).

Spirituality

Metaphysical and spiritual processes, "the desire to situate birth within realms of meaning beyond the biological act itself" (Klassen 2001), historically played a defining role in some midwives' work, personal, and community identities. Several women explained how these elements, once valued, were later scorned in the move to professionalization, and how they were urged to suppress or abandon their more public displays of spirituality.

One woman expressed her belief that "there is a connection between midwives, mothers, birth, and the universe" that was not being honoured in the move to professionalization. She felt that her faith in such a connection had created an impediment to becoming registered:

> I think that's why I haven't been able to make it so far and if I continue not to be able to make it that is why. I think that the realm of experience and that realm of practice has been a priori dismissed. It does not belong. It does not exist. You must not talk about it. You can pay lip service to such things as dealing with the "whole woman" – you know, her physical, social, and psychological needs – but you can't talk about her spirituality any more because what is that? Well, it may mean getting together with a bunch of women and chanting around the fireplace but anything further than that we don't want to talk about. (Interview no. 18)

In an astute analysis of the conflict between the scientific/rational model of childbearing and "spiritual midwifery," she added:

> I think the midwives and the folks who bought into this whole thing, they bought into this idea that if you couch things in physical terms and if you couch things in measurable, repeatable, verifiable – you know the mythology

of the scientific method – that then they are controllable, they are predictable, they are dealable with and you can avoid any situation that is too scary ... When you start to admit that there are forces at work other than the purely physical and that such forces are not subject to human control and prediction then you do threaten that [rational] structure. (Interview no. 18)

Another woman recalled being admonished by elite midwives in the prelegislation period "not to talk at all on media about spiritual concerns ... or the spiritual walk of midwifery" (Interview no. 17). She compared this attitude and the disciplinary atmosphere of Ontario to another province where she had worked as a midwife: "In [that province], you don't have elite groups going off and having their retreats. Everybody goes off to have a retreat all together. And we're allowed to light candles and put pictures on the floor about how we see our relationship with the universe at the moment. And we allow ourselves to talk about how we're feeling before we get into the meeting. We're allowed to talk quite freely and it's a different culture."

Rituals such as those described above became, in the years just prior to legalization, the object of public mockery in the midwifery community. In a recent master's thesis, Ontario midwife Betty-Anne Daviss (1999, 69) described how informants in her study remembered an incident when spiritual rituals once common among Ontario midwives were publicly derided: "Holding of hands had long been ruled out and considered inappropriate behaviour among professional midwives in the province ... At an AGM of the AOM in 1990, for instance a skit in which some midwives at a meeting pass a rock around a circle was remembered by some interviewees as a way of ridiculing such rituals. It was also considered a subtle means of deterring anyone from suggesting such goings-on in the future."

If, as Jane Flax (1993, 42) posits, science is a "privileged practice within modern knowledge/power systems," it is unimaginable that the struggle to constitute women as rational humanist subjects in the eyes of the state could be won (in the case of midwifery) through claims to a spiritual rather than a rational and scientific epistemology. Consequently, it should not be surprising that the "starry-eyed earth mother" – a figure of spiritual excess – was identified within the midwifery movement as an impediment to public confidence in the new profession and to its acceptance within the scientific community. The disciplining, then, of those who clung to an earlier vision of the midwife – one in which scientific and metaphysical knowledge existed in continual tension – seemed an urgent necessity.

Dress and Appearance

Alexandra Warwick and Dani Cavallaro (1998, xvi) argue that "dress acts as a daily reminder of our dependence on margins and boundaries for the purposes of self-construction." Wearing the "yellow socks and Birkenstock sandals" cited in the opening epigraph situated a midwife on the wrong side of the respectability/degeneracy divide. Admonitions about the necessity of presenting a respectable appearance in order to, as one midwife put it, "get away from the image of the hippie midwife, the spiritual midwife, the midwife who doesn't look like a nurse-practitioner" (Interview no. 17) reminded midwives regularly about the counterculture "other" against whom new midwifery identities needed to be constituted. Several of the women interviewed spoke at length about expectations around appearance during the preregistration period. One midwife, in a quote that recognizes implicitly the role of dress in producing subjectivity through a linking of the individual to a collectivity, remembered a discussion that flagged the drawbacks of conducting an interview with the press in one's home because "the background ... would look too 'crunchy granola,' so you'd have to dress in a certain way. There was an incredible amount of stuff about image ... I don't want to play little games like that, but it's politically very smart, of course, because then one has a certain image and one can become part of the other group because one has the image of that group" (Interview no. 20). Another woman related her own comical and largely ineffectual efforts to adopt a more respectable appearance in the years before legalization: "There was a joke along for a while where people would come out of a media event and go, 'I looked just like a nurse-midwife!' So I got a perm and I looked like a cross between Shirley Temple and an English judge – and I looked *more* like a hippie!" (Interview no. 17).

For these and other white women in the midwifery movement, presenting a respectable appearance was as easy as changing their wardrobe or hairdo. If the offending markers could be abandoned, then presumably their bodies could fade back into what Judith Butler (2000, 59) has called the "taken-for-granted visual field" in which able white bodies appear unremarkable. Bodies of colour and disabled bodies can never occupy this default position of invisibility, which raises important questions about who can be (literally) seen as a respectable midwifery subject.

Constructing Respectable Midwives in the Midwifery Education Program

Between 1993 and 1997, 2,475 people applied for admission to approximately 175 spaces in the baccalaureate-granting Midwifery Education Program (MEP) offered in three Ontario universities: Ryerson Polytechnic University in Toronto, Laurentian University in Sudbury, and McMaster University in Hamilton (Stewart and Pong 1998). Students have been remarkably homogeneous in terms of their demographic characteristics. They are uniformly female; approximately half are married; a large majority have children; their ages ranged, on the average from twenty-eight to thirty-three; they are overwhelmingly native English speakers; and they have increasingly entered the MEP having already earned a postsecondary diploma, with 79 percent of the 1996 student population bringing with them a previous university degree (Stewart and Pong 1997, 14). Statistics have not been collected related to applicants' or students' race and/or ethnicity, but one trend that *has* been documented is a consistent decline in the proportion of midwifery aspirants whose mother tongue was neither English nor French. Applications from this group dropped from 15 percent in the 1993 cohort to 6.8 percent in the 1997 cohort (Stewart and Pong 1998, 9). Anecdotal evidence I collected about the 1993-97 classes of MEP participants, as well as more recent research (Bailey 2002) indicates that the midwifery student body has been overwhelmingly composed of white women.

Many of the students who participated, between 1993 and 1998, in the Humber College/Women's College Hospital Childbirth Educators Multidiscipline Certificate Program had enrolled in the course to maximize their chances of being selected for the Midwifery Education Program. Sixteen certified childbirth educators (not all from the HC/WCH program) were admitted to the MEP between 1993 and 1996 (Stewart and Pong 1997, 25), indicating that it was a valued credential. With only one out of every fifteen applicants being accepted into the MEP, there was vigorous speculation about the qualities and experience being sought by the admissions committees. Women in the childbirth educators program that I taught often discussed this, and they eagerly questioned former students who had been accepted to the MEP when they visited the classroom as guest lecturers. I read and critiqued many MEP application letters for my students, and they frequently phoned me to tell me how they had fared in the admissions process. Those who had gained coveted interviews spoke of the careful attention they paid to demonstrating a generally normative appearance and to censoring their responses to interviewers' questions so as to communicate neither too radical nor too conservative a political sensibility. While presentation of a highly normative self is an efficacious strategy for those seeking to gain admission to prestigious human services professions, and most of us engage in such practices daily, the accounts I was hearing suggested that an extraordinary disciplinarity was in evidence within the MEP. Stories from those who were accepted to the program seemed to confirm this perception and the anger of some students was palpable. Expecting a liberal, even liberatory space, a "sort of bubble, a nice happy place" (Interview no. 38), students were frustrated and disappointed by what they encountered. Subsequent interviews that I conducted with eleven midwifery students suggested that the normalizing impulse in the MEP, notably in relation to gender, sexuality, ability, spirituality, class, and, of course, race, has led some students to engage in a rigorous policing of the self. So intense had the experience been for one student of colour who felt forced to dissimulate that she told me, "When I get through this program, then I'm going to be myself" (Interview no. 41). This sentiment was frequently articulated by other students.

Dressing like "Avon Ladies": Appearance Norms as a Microstrategy of Power

Midwifery students I interviewed offered narratives that provided a glimpse into the microstrategies of power that Foucault described in *Discipline and Punish* (1979). Such strategies are not strictly coercive, but work through the setting of norms embedded in "ostensibly beneficent and scientific forms of knowledge" (McNay 1994, 95). The human body is the ultimate target of such strategies, and perhaps nowhere is their disciplinary reach more palpable than in their shaping of the way the body is publicly presented. Seen as critical to public acceptance and therefore to midwifery's liberatory agenda of providing more childbearing options for women, the adoption of a normative bodily appearance seems a rational choice rather than an effect of power. However, as Warwick and Cavallaro (1998) argue, dress is a "complex transfer point of power relations" and has an important role in both discipline and transgression. Dress and grooming are sites where gender, race, and sexuality are coded, often in and through one another. For midwifery students, messages on how to dress, coif, and groom themselves served as reminders that for the fragile profession the boundary between respectability and degeneracy was not yet secure and that transgressive appearance had the power to link midwives to any number of socially marginal groups. I have at least two concerns with this form of disciplinarity: (1) for members of marginalized groups who use clothing or other forms of body decoration as a way of marking identity, a requirement to adopt a "normalized" appearance makes it difficult to connect with other group members; and (2) defaulting into the taken-for-granted visual field can be successful only for those not corporeally marked by their difference. If, as one student of colour was told when she began the MEP, the goal was for midwifery students to look like "Avon ladies" – meaning, I presume, an idealized vision of a heterosexual white suburban woman – then normative midwifery subjecthood was not available to those who could never cram themselves into its narrow confines. As the student quoted above went on to note, "If you're a racialized person, this is like you're way out on the edge of acceptability to begin with. It's like Avon ladies don't look like me to begin with" (Interview no. 42).

All the students interviewed referred to a lecture delineating the bounds of acceptable dress that they received in the early part of their midwifery training.[18] While no one actually undertook to define what respectable apparel consisted of, they did know what was unacceptable (T-shirts, leather jackets, jeans with holes and rips, and so on), which is to say clothes identified with youth or sexual subcultures. A student who had grown up in poverty recalled that the lecture linked dress and respectability indelibly in her mind: "We had to be 'ambassadors of the profession.' I remember this vividly because it was part of the dress code thing and was horrible, a horrible talk" (Interview no. 43). The effect of such a prescription can be seen in students' constant preoccupation with how they were dressed both in the classroom and in the hospital, where scrutiny by doctors and nurses was expected and normative appearance took on greater significance. A woman nearing the end of her program remarked, "We've got to be presentable, basically to these white men who are obstetricians" (Interview no. 42). Another student said that being on call forced her to think about how she dressed at all times. "It's one of my worst fears," she said. "I'm always afraid, like in the back of my mind every morning, if I get paged right now and I got to the hospital is someone going to go, 'She's a midwifery student? She looks like shit. She looks like a hippie!'" (Interview no. 33). For another student, a call from the hospital sent her running to "get my makeup and my perfume on at like three in the morning" (Interview no. 41). For yet another student, the dress code loomed large in her daily decision about what to wear, which was complicated, in turn, by her hesitation, as a lesbian, to adopt a style of dress that might mark her as excessive or invoke a homophobic response from clients:

So, like, I won't wear, I think I did once, at the beginning of the year, I was really nervous about the whole thing ... but I won't wear, like I have some really, really ripped-up jeans and I'm afraid to wear them to school. I am! I think that, like, especially being the lesbian, that makes it worse right? So I don't wear my ripped jeans to school ... I do have a sweater that has a big rip in the elbows, it's about ten years old and I love that sweater. I've seen [a midwifery professor] staring at my elbows when I'm wearing it and I'm thinking, "What is she thinking?" Anyway, so when I have a client visit, I always think "Okay, what am I going to wear today?" cause I'm going to visit a client today. I think like that. I do think that as a student I have to try harder to be more sort of mainstreamy presentable because these women can, for any fucking reason in the world, decide not to have me at their birth. (Interview no. 35)

Students were also warned away from forms of self-presentation that were not normatively feminine or that signalled an unconventional sexual identity, such as displaying unshaven legs or underarms. For some students, these proscriptions represented the limits of tolerability and became loci of resistance. One student who took particular offence to the dress code was reported to have shaved her head the night before her scheduled appearance as a student representative at a public "midwifery information night." One interviewee believed that this student, who was subsequently chastised by an MEP faculty member, had done it to "let everybody know that *she* was in the program and had no hair, kind of thing" (Interview no. 39). For this student, a lesbian, shaving her head constituted an act of resistance to the imperative to remain unmarked and therefore respectable. But it also raised a "subcultural flag" (Silverman 1986, 147) that allowed her to signal the existence of what had been rendered unthinkable: the possibility (however risky) of simultaneously occupying the discursive space of midwife *and* lesbian.

Sexuality and Reproductive Identities in the MEP

Like the student who shaved her head in protest, students I interviewed had a strong sense of which sexual and reproductive identities were considered to be appropriate for "ambassadors of the profession." During the focus group that I conducted with six midwifery students, they spontaneously ranked sexual and reproductive identities from most to least acceptable, reflecting a strong perception that homosexual and bisexual identities were only marginally acceptable within the MEP.

Interviewee no. 33: Definitely children, definitely.

Interviewee no. 34: You see the best ... the thing to do is to be married with children. The next best thing to do is to be in a heterosexual relationship with a partner.

Interviewee no. 33: And then "used to be in a heterosexual relationship."

Interviewee no. 34: Yeah, there's sort of that hierarchy.

Interviewee no. 41: Definitely not a chosen single mother for sure.

Interviewee no. 34: A chosen single mother is the worst, you know. A lesbian partner is okay.

Interviewee no. 41: Maybe but ...

Interviewee no. 34: Single lesbian is ...

Interviewee no. 41: And to like be someone without children is like "Well, you're aspiring to have children, so it's okay." If you said you didn't know if you wanted to have children, it's like "'What the hell are you doing here?'"

Interviewee no. 32: There are real ideas about when you should be having your children.

All: Yeah, totally.

Occupying the hybrid space of midwife *and* lesbian has presented a particular challenge for students who must make daily choices about disclosing aspects of their sexual identities. As it did with other marginalized groups, Ontario midwifery invoked its own respectability by positioning lesbians as available for rescue (from heterosexist medicine) through midwives' provision of sensitive care, including "interpreting lesbian culture to the hospital staff" (Ford 1992, 5). No mention is made of the role of lesbian midwives nor of the complications they might face as practitioners in a homophobic medical/social environment. The "lesbian baby boom" notwithstanding, lesbian midwives face numerous issues when they negotiate their relationship to childbearing from the (heteronormative) categorical space of non-reproducers (Herman 1996, 88). I believe that this topic, beyond the scope of this research, awaits serious exploration.[19] I can address here only the problematic negotiations of identity that lesbian and bisexual students in the MEP shared with me, and their relation to the bending of midwifery bodies toward normativity.

. Eve Kosofsky Sedgwick has argued that for most gay men and lesbians, silence, intermittently imposed and broken in relation to the discursive context in which it is deployed, continues to be a fundamental feature of social life. "There can be few gay people," Sedgwick (1990, 68) maintains, "however courageous and forthright by habit, however fortunate in the support of their immediate communities in whose lives the closet is not a shaping presence." For four students interviewed here who identified as lesbian or bisexual, life as a student midwife involved a concerted closeting in relationship to clients and frequent reminders by other students of the improbability of the subject position "lesbian midwife."

While two of the students I spoke with either self-identified as lesbians on the application to the MEP or did so in their interviews, both knew several other lesbian women who had not. One woman hesitated about being "out" in her application but felt that being closeted would prevent her from displaying her organizational experience, much of which had been gained during her years of queer activism. "I hemmed and hawed about that for a couple of years before I applied and decided I had to do it because I don't know how to talk about all my accomplishments without talking about all my queer stuff" (Interview no. 35). She was prepared, however, if denied admission, to submit a subsequent application in which she would conceal her sexuality.

Another lesbian student described the circumscribed nature of being out in the MEP. It was possible for her and others to self-identify privately, but they still encountered homophobic comments from colleagues. Acknowledging that there is some measure of tolerance for lesbian students, this student linked the closeting of lesbian educators with the impossibility of a public subjectivity in which the identities "lesbian" and "midwife" are intertwined and the creation of an atmosphere in which homophobic comments are voiced with seeming impunity:

There's a lot of queer people in this program. But not in an out way. Like, we acknowledge it on a personal level and in small groups you can also talk about it. It's not completely closeted. But knowing that your professors are queer and never talk about it and knowing that there have been instances in midwifery where people have said, "I don't know, like if you can be a lesbian and a midwife." Knowing students who were talking about a program called Dykes and Tykes for lesbian mothers and their children and they say, "Dykes and Tykes! What's going on? When I had kids it was Moms and Tots." (Interview no. 41)

Women also described relationships with clients in which they felt closeting was mandatory. In the quotation below, a midwifery student describes an awkward incident with a client:

I was leaving her and at the corner she was saying, "Do you have a babysitter? If I called you in the middle of the night, do you have a babysitter?" I said, "Oh, no, I don't have a babysitter." She says, "I was talking to your nanny" and it was a friend of mine who's British! And I said, "I don't have a nanny." And she said, "But who's going to look after ..." I said, "I don't have a babysitter." She said, "Who'll look after your son?" And I said, "I live with someone and we look after our son together." But I wasn't about to come out, right? 'Cause I thought, "This woman's a Christian, and she's not somebody I'm going to come out to and I feel fine about that." I don't feel like I have to and I don't feel like I'm diminished." (Interview no. 37)

Such encounters are everyday occurrences for gay and lesbian people, and the student quoted above was not personally offended by the client's presumption of her heterosexuality. The question here is, to what degree a normative image for the midwifery profession contributes to the student's burden of silence. As I have stated above, the subject position "lesbian midwife," a distinct interruption of the profession's current image, is simply not available within public discourse in Canada.

In the United States, however, midwife Anne Frye has conducted a decades-long struggle, within the highly heteronormative US direct-entry midwifery movement, to not only create a discursive space for the lesbian midwife but to intervene in everyday assumptions about sexual orientation. Once her voice was constituted as authoritative, Frye used her visible presence to change the public discourse and to interrupt the movement's complicity in relations of domination:

When people see that the people they work with, and who take care of them at any level – their service people, their medical care providers, their sons and daughters, their aunts and uncles – are the very same people that are lesbians and gays, then it puts it into an entirely different context and makes it harder for lesbians and gays to be the "other weird people."

I work for predominantly heterosexual women – and it is a calling, not a nine-to-five job. So to feel that some of those same women would ostracize or condemn me for who I am is very intense and makes me that much more committed to be out as a lesbian ... I chose to come out into the midwifery community after I had made a name for myself with my work as a recognized writer and speaker. Because I thought that with people knowing who I was and then adding to that my being a lesbian would make it harder for them to reject me. And hopefully my coming out would create more safety for other midwives who want to come out. I want to make sure on an organizational level that we don't support the intrinsic homophobia in our culture. (Quoted in Chester 1997, 122)

The issues around closeting are complex and involve, among other things, the constant struggle to weigh the very real potential consequences (including physical violence) of being out, with the public and private benefits of refusing the closet. In one recent Canadian study, nearly 12 percent of those sampled in an urban area said they would refuse to be treated by a gay, lesbian, or bisexual physician (Druzinet et al., quoted in Beagan 1998, 46). The absence of a public discourse in which midwifery identities are multiple seemed to contribute to lesbian and bisexual students' decisions to remain closeted or largely circumspect in their relations with other students, with most clients, and with some midwives who served as their clinical preceptors in the field. What must be acknowledged is how the impulse to create respectable "ambassadors of the profession" has required a complicitous relationship with heterosexual norms.

Class and Family Normativity

In terms of deportment and access to material resources, students described the tyranny of a middle-class norm in the Midwifery Education Program and their own reticence to be seen to fall outside of its confines. One student described her reluctance to challenge assumptions within the program because she would then be, in her words, "outed" as a poor person:

I have come to this program, this state in my life, with a lot of baggage about not having money, about surviving on welfare. It's not something I openly discuss or talk about. I get upset when people assume we can afford books, we can afford tuition, no one questions. When I have questions about OSAP [Ontario Student Assistance Program], like the next year, we're going to struggle, I don't know how we're going to do it, and I police myself. I haven't called other students to ask how they cope. I haven't talked to my course advisor on how people cope. I've been very reluctant to ... I feel

I'm outing myself as a poor person. I've survived all my life as a poor person. I've got great survival skills; I could probably share them with other people, but I don't feel like it's understood. I don't feel it's respected. We're told at the beginning, when you were sent your offer of admission, you were told that it was going to be expensive and you couldn't have a job and you had to survive and you had to have a car. And I thought, so basically, I thought we were told, "If you're poor, forget about it. You should drop out now." (Interview no. 43)

Another student conceded that when it came to explaining in their MEP applications how they would support themselves during the segments of the program where they were not allowed to have outside jobs, students "all lie about that. I realize we have more money than some people. We at least can fake it, right?" (Interview no. 35).

"Faking it" for some students involved relying on the advantages conferred by whiteness. For working-class women, whiteness allowed middle-class identities to be performed through a mimicking of bourgeois behaviour and appearance standards. A retreat into the taken-for-granted visual field of whiteness was available if markers of poverty were concealed or erased. One woman, who clearly grasps how women positioned subordinately in relation to class may use race privilege to gain a "toehold on respectability" (Fellows and Razack 1998), explained how this process works: "I, as someone who grew up *really* poor, like we were dirt poor and I have been thinking more about that too. How class fits into my world and how white privilege has been part of my being able to get through fine, like kind of. Like you just kind of meander your way through and you cut your nails, you clean your nails before an interview, you know you put caps on your teeth or something. But it can be done" (Interview no. 37).

For some of the students, "middle class" denoted not only access to resources and knowing how to comport and present the self in a respectable manner, it involved being able to claim a family of origin free from emotional upheaval of any kind. One student claimed that what she was careful not to disclose in the context of the MEP was "my fucked-up life. Like I feel that everyone in the program comes from or appears to come from this really white middle-class very 'family' background. And I have none of that ... I hide so many things, like a sibling dying when I was a child and my father dying, in terms of a lot of that stuff. It's like, oh my God, I can't be a superwoman and a good professional if I've had this sort of screwed-up life" (Interview no. 41). This student argued cannily in her application questionnaire that because of her unsettled family history she possessed extraordinarily good stress-management skills. While this may or may not have worried the admissions committee, it did not prevent them from offering her a place in the MEP. Another student, however, believed that admitting to a chaotic upbringing may have jeopardized her previous unsuccessful applications and she chose to sanitize her final application, which was successful. "By the time I wrote a questionnaire that got me interviewed," she told me, "none of that was in there any more" (Interview no. 33). Whether or not admissions committees judge applicants on these bases is immaterial. The simple perception of the norm is adequate to produce a policing of bodies and a rewriting of personal histories that reinscribe economic and emotional normativity as indispensable elements of respectability. In this process, however, those who are seen as unworthy of inclusion in the new midwifery profession resurface in the figure of the needy "other" who is available for rescue and whose proximity and otherness help define the dominant midwifery subject. One student described this process when she recalled an exercise conducted in a workshop that dealt with identities:

> You were allowed to create your own categories for identity and somebody had written down "survivors of violence" or something. And tons of people went ... maybe fifteen or twenty people out of a group of thirty wrote down, just wrote ticks that they would ... that that's where they would place their identity. And yet when we ever do workshops, it's all with the perspective of "these poor women who've been battered by their husbands, these poor women who are divorced, these poor women were abused as children, these poor women ..." There's never any mention that somehow that might have been your experience. (Interview no. 34)

The subject who can be universalized is most desirable within the MEP. One student, a woman who identifies as working class, recalled that in her first (unsuccessful) application she spoke from her specific class identity and as a marginalized person. Deeming such an approach inefficacious, she adopted a different strategy in the following year's application: "The next year that I applied, instead of talking a lot about 'this is who I am' and 'this is why I have this experience,' and 'I very personally identify with these issues as well as my professional experience,' I very much focused on my professional, you know, 'I am a professional, I work with these "other" women.' And it was very the 'other.' ... My tone was more as a service delivery person and not from my own experience" (Interview no. 43).

Disability

In an environment in which the able body is constructed as normal through its relationship to an environment that accommodates only ableness, disability becomes an "intense, extravagant, and problematic embodiment" (Thomson 1997, 283). Wishing to avoid being viewed as inherently problematic, some students chose to conceal their disabilities in their application questionnaires to the MEP. One woman who suffers from an emotional

disorder had not disclosed her disability to other MEP students before doing so in the group interview conducted for this study. She had remained
silent, she related, "because it's so taboo, first of all, in society. And second
of all, it's not seen as a disability issue. It seems like you're screwed up"
(Interview no. 41). A second woman, whose disability is intermittently visible depending on its severity at the time, made a conscious decision not to
flag her physical limitations on her application. Once admitted to the program, she policed herself constantly to contain any nuance of vulnerability.
While she has found the faculty generally supportive, any admission of
weakness causes her capability to be questioned:

> There have been instances where I have said, "I can't do this" or "I want to
> do this earlier rather than later because I'm in pain," or whatever. And the
> response is, "Well, are you sure you can be a midwife? What are you going
> to do when you're out there practising?" I'm not in practice right now, I'm
> in school and writing an exam. That's not the issue. And when I go into
> placement I always feel extra pressure. I can't be the one at the birth saying
> "I'm tired" or I can't be the one taking a day off sick. Because if I take a day
> off sick, I might really be sick! But if I say it, it might be because I'm disabled
> and therefore I won't be a good midwife. (Interview no. 39)

This student has found her physical capacities questioned unrelentingly
and her body constantly an object of interest and comparison. Even her
right to reproduce was seen as an appropriate topic for interrogation: "I've
had students say to me, 'How do you know it was okay for you to have kids?
Do you know what you *did* to the next generation?' (in relation to my not
being able to conceive instantly and having a disability and who knows
what I've passed on to my son). I was sort of floored that it was okay for her
to say that. But it *was* okay" (Interview no. 39). The one student who has
not been able to conceal her disability believes that her admission to the
MEP was judged by other students to have been based not on her suitability
for the program, but rather on her being an "equity admission." In an environment in which respectability needed constant securing through the
normalization of bodies, the presence of the disabled body – unavailable for
universalization and normalization – could only be understood to have been
included through coercion.

Spirituality
Counterculture spirituality was a mark of excess for prelegislation midwives,
and for the students I interviewed, even affiliations with relatively dominant religious institutions appeared to threaten their suitability as midwives.
One student, a former member of a religious order, described having the

Christian identity she carefully hid for a year and half in the MEP inadvertently discovered during another student's visit to her home:

> B was at my house and looked at my fridge and went, "Are you a Christian?" ... I mean, we were in the program for a year and half and [she says], "You're a Christian? You were a nun!" And yeah, I don't know anyone else in the program who's an ex-nun and so that's a big piece, all the religious stuff. I have to be really, really careful about the religious stuff. All the stereotypes that go around Christian ... and so to be careful about what you say because of all the stereotypes ... I think one piece of that is, I'm not quite sure how to say it, but the things that Christians have done and whatever it is. I mean the stereotypes around their position on homosexuality, on abortion, their position on being judgmental, whatever ... That you can't be a feminist and be a Christian. You can't be a lesbian and be a Christian. You can't be all that sort of stuff, I think, is one piece. (Interview no. 34)

While this student's lived experience confirms that one can simultaneously embrace Christian and feminist beliefs, there is no discursive space in which to occupy these positions simultaneously within the MEP. Her only recourse is silence. The anti-abortion and antihomosexual doctrines and politics of the Catholic Church, and the relative invisibility of oppositional voices within it, make it more difficult to forge complex subject positions between Catholic affiliation and other forms of identity. However, it is not just Catholicism that has brought students' rationality and ability to be universalized into question. One woman with strong Protestant affiliations agreed that spirituality was viewed as incompatible with midwifery identity and said that she had kept silent about her own affiliations and beliefs. Although she was granted permission, she was still questioned vigorously about her plans to take a course in a divinity school. She was advised by one student not to speak openly about the course: "And it was like, 'I'm not sure exactly why I'm not supposed to say that.' Because it's not related to midwifery? [...] Or because I'll go off and ... I don't know ... become ordained instead of practising as a midwife? I don't know, but this really felt like something I couldn't talk about" (Interview no. 32).

These narratives suggest that midwifery students envisioned a normative midwifery subject and strived to conform in a number of ways. The tyranny of the norm operated in the MEP to discipline students' bodies and to produce relatively docile and respectable "ambassadors of the profession." However, whatever their positioning at other axes of difference, white students and students of colour are regulated differently by this process. Kate Davy (1995, 9) has succinctly summarized how such regulation works: "Played out in the politics of respectability, whiteness becomes the dynamic that underpins a process of racialization that feeds privilege to all whites, so to speak, without letting all white people sit at the table. Those middle-class people of color invited to sit at the table are bequeathed a status that is always already only honorary, contingent, itinerant, and temporary." For those who could, assuming the default position of whiteness in the "taken-for-granted visual field" conferred a level of respectability and a modicum of protection from unrelenting scrutiny. Consequently, most lesbian students, who, indisputably, were forced to observe their own codes of silence and were required routinely to engage in soul-numbing performances of heterosexual normativity, could expect a meal, if not a banquet, at the table of whiteness and at least had a critical mass of other lesbian students with whom they could identify. The option to "pass," notes Dana Takagi (1996, 247), is not available to racialized minority people: "We do not think in advance about whether or not to present ourselves as 'Asian American,' rather that is an identification that is worn by us, whether we like it or not, and which is easily read off of us by others." Consequently, for racialized minority people, historical discourses of difference arise unrelentingly in the face-to-face encounters with whites that are the stuff of everyday life. Students of colour, then, found themselves renegotiating their place at the midwifery table on a daily basis.

Students of Colour in the Midwifery Education Program

Three of the students interviewed self-identified as women of colour and reported that their experiences in the MEP had been marked intermittently by overt and covert racist incidents, by a sense of either invisibility or voyeuristic display, and by constant feelings of isolation. While there were positive aspects to their participation in the MEP, and not all students of colour would offer such narratives, these are the experiences that those I interviewed chose to speak about when I posed the question "How have you policed yourself in the midwifery education program?"[20] The critical relationship between silence and survival was a constant theme for these women. They were silent in order to avoid confrontation during racist incidents, silenced and imperilled because of the absence of a community of equally positioned speakers, and silent within their communities of origin because they are unable to disclose that they were not the "pioneers" within the midwifery program they were thought to be. The double bind of silence was described by one woman thus: "I felt that I was betraying my own community, betraying myself by my silence, and still I struggle with that, but I know that I wouldn't have got through if I hadn't been silent" (Interview no. 42).

These students were interviewed at different stages in their programs and had had varying degrees of contact with midwifery preceptors and clients. These factors had an impact on the breadth of their experiences and therefore upon the range and number of instances of racism they encountered. Attention must be directed as well to the fact that interview material from one student of colour was collected in the context of a group interview in which the rest of the participants, including myself, were white. She spoke fairly openly about racism and other matters to this politically sophisticated group (and to me as the avowedly antiracist researcher and as someone known to her outside of this context), but she probably also left much unsaid. In retrospect, I can see the error in conducting a racially mixed focus group, even when the participants appear to enjoy a modicum of trust. This is a perfect example of how (even well-intentioned) white women are regulated to overlook the difference that race makes. Because of this methodological limitation, and because she shared interview time with five other women, this woman is perhaps less fully represented here than other students of colour who were interviewed individually. Their voices, consequently, dominate this section. The woman who was closest to finishing – only weeks away at the time of our interview – recalled a larger number of overtly racist incidents than did the other two women. She also spoke frequently about the potential consequences of confronting racism directly when its source was midwifery preceptors who had the power to impede a student's completion of her program. The other two women had not yet had extended contact with preceptors and clients.

In the narratives of the two students of colour who were interviewed separately, silence as a condition and a consequence of survival appears frequently. In addition, both women use metaphors of death and dying to describe the consequences of speech. For one student, to speak out is "suicide," and another student longed for a time when she would find the strength to speak freely; otherwise, she lamented, she would become a "walking dead person." That parts of the self have, for these women, been violently excised in the process of becoming a midwife must be acknowledged. I am quoting these students at length because such testimonies have not been part of the public discourse about midwifery, at least not among white people, and so that I might avoid the epistemic violence that would be enacted if I were to uncouple the recounting of the racist incident from the emotional context of its telling:

> It would just be suicide for me to really talk about issues that are important to me as a woman of colour and my experience and what I perceive as important to the birthing community who experience things as I do ... It was always confirmed to me that I had to be very careful that there was no place for the diversity of experience to be shared ... So well, I guess the thing that I've learned in my life is that in order to get through I've got to be silent because if I really speak my mind ... and it's not about speaking my mind out of anger and resentment, its out of working for change ... It's not

just "oh, I'm angry at white women because whatever," but that I have a voice that ... and it's presumed or assumed or perceived that my voice or needs are the same as white women's and it's not ... I would definitely fear really expressing who I am and the repercussions at this point because ... and certainly throughout the program ... because I was vulnerable. I had preceptors who were brutal, who put me through hell. So I was just "yes sir, yes ma'am, no ma'am" all the way through. And that was the only way I was going to get through. (Interview no. 42)

Within the universalizing bosom of midwifery, this woman is tolerated only if she does not name the power that renders her silent. To do so would cause her to be "guilty of that most wretched of native sins – ingratitude" (Razack 2000, 42). The assumption, as she states above, is that she does not have sensibilities that differ in any way from white women's, so articulating racist sentiments in her presence is not perceived as injurious:

When you silence yourself then you hear things more because people assume you'll never say anything. And you just hear things more and people say things even more cause they don't see you at all ... One of the midwives I was with was talking to a client and they were talking about, I think it was abortion ... And the midwife, who was against abortion, actually talked about ... well, she sort of identified with the woman 'cause she was a Christian too, and the woman had said, "Well, you know I don't believe in it, but I accept the people that I work with and their choices, dah, dah, dah." And then the midwife went on to say, "Yeah, well, I've worked with all sorts of people. I've worked with ..." And she ... I forget the tone, but it was like the tone, too, that was major, but she said how she had worked ... she had even worked with lesbians. No, she had even worked with *a* lesbian and that she had even worked with heathens in [a southern continent]. And [laughter] I'm standing right there and I have a name [associated with that continent]. I'm not ... I don't associate myself as a Christian, although I have some Christian background. Anyway so it goes over her head; she has no idea what she is saying. (Interview no. 42)

Relaying another instance of her invisibility, this woman spoke about an incident with a client:

And there have been clients, too, that have said things. Like the little cap on the baby's head: "Oh, he looks like he's one of the grand ..." I don't know what the leaders are of the Ku Klux Klan. But "one of the grand so and so's of the Ku Klux Klan, doesn't he?" And you know, things like that, and there I am standing right there and they smile at me – they think that I think it's cute, too. And I just carry on because I neither have the power in that environment or I don't know what you need to address those things. But it's just like I'm trying to get through this day, you know. (Interview no. 42)

Silencing also occurs when one is compelled to speak inauthentically and is, as the student quoted below describes poignantly, a soul-destroying imperative. It is only the promise of future independence and credibility that sustains hope:

I'm quite silent, very silent, I don't say a word. And when things come up, even if ... yeah, like I don't take the opportunity to ... like there's a couple of times at the [midwifery] practice that I'm at where it just came up that the way people were talking – that I could say something about cultural sensitivity. I try not to go into the whole thing not trusting, 'cause of course there are wonderful surprises wherever you are. But comments like, I've heard at my practice, she mentioned a nurse, "It was that Chinese girl and she was awful." She was talking about a nurse. And I thought, like there's just constant things that remind me that people aren't aware of their own racism. They aren't. I don't see an openness and I don't see support.

The environment is quietly or passively hostile to women of colour speaking about their experiences. Of course, we could speak about our experiences in an apologetic way, in a multicultural, smooth, kind of "sugar on top" way. Of course, that would be loved 'cause that would help midwifery in Ontario feel good about itself. But for women of colour to speak honestly about our direct experiences with other midwives, with the system of midwifery, with the history of midwifery, the way midwives are perceived in other countries, the way women of colour are perceived – I just don't see that I can do that. And it's a horrible place to be in, I tell you, it feels like you're in a desert.

But I just keep thinking that I'm going to get to a place where I'm going to be able to be ... hang on to a strong tree or stand like a strong tree and speak my mind. And I'm going to be, that's what I want to do. That's the only way I can live, otherwise I'm a walking dead person. (Interview no. 43)

One form of silencing involves not having access to communities of discourse where experiences of racism could be openly discussed and others could be counted on for support in raising issues. In another "life and death" metaphor, one woman claimed, "It's suicide if you do something, if you speak up in isolation. You'll be brutalized; you're just like a duck" (Interview no. 42). She described how difficult it was to make contact with other women of colour, not only because they were scarce, but also because the heavy workload made extracurricular involvements practically impossible. When she did manage to speak with another woman of colour, she related that "both of us were almost moved to tears that we had never spoken about these things. But when we did it was just so clear to both of us, you know, the oppressiveness of it all and the contradictions of it all, and the need to work within our own communities."

For another woman, a lesbian of colour, the absence of other students of colour made disclosing her sexuality practically unthinkable: "I remember ... arriving in Sudbury [for the 'intensive' midwifery introduction for new MEP entrants] and my sister and my girlfriend dropping me off and them looking into the room and just looking at me and going, 'Oh, my God.' 'Cause it was entirely white and it was very straight looking. And I walked in and said, 'I'm the only dyke,' and I'm not ... they know I'm brown, I'm not going to tell them that I'm a dyke!" (Interview no. 41). Unwilling to imperil the respectability available to her through her middle-class status, this woman chose not to identify herself immediately as a lesbian. As Kate Davy (1995, 10) argues, it is only white women who can "demand the right to be 'bad' without reinscribing an already naturalized deviance."

Self-imposed silence is a doubled-edged sword. For one student, a reticence to speak about race issues during her clinical placements constituted a survival strategy. However, it also foreclosed the possibility of communicating with clients of colour on issues that fell beyond the bounds of white-defined midwifery practice. She reflected with regret upon how her survival strategies in a racist environment caused her to impose silence on other women of colour:

It's interesting 'cause a sad thing about it is that I guess I don't ... you don't realize it when you silence yourself, but you're not only silencing yourself in order to cope with white women who are hostile to your identity. But in doing that I think that I also, without realizing it, may silence other women of colour who come in my care, because I'm so quiet about that aspect of who we are. Yeah, so that's kind of sad. It took me aback when I was at a birth with a woman of colour and she asked me directly, like one day ... well, two things. One day she asked me directly, she said – 'cause she was dealing with death, her baby had died – and she asked me directly, "How in _____ culture do they deal with death?" She was of _____ descent and she really wanted to know more about her cultural tradition in that and wanted to explore that with me. And another day we just ended up talking about race and I never, ever bring these things up because I have no – partly because I'm getting accustomed to being silent and partly because I don't know what the reactions are going to be: if I'm not in a safe place, if there was negative reactions. And so I've been sort of taken aback when it's brought up because it makes me realize that I probably give less opportunity for it to be brought up because I'm so much in a mode of silencing that aspect of myself. And in turn, [I'm] probably indirectly silencing that aspect of other women of colour. So it's participating in it all. And that's the really sad aspect of it. (Interview no. 42)

The student quoted above did not speak of racism to other racialized minority people because she felt that if she, as the "model minority student," discussed her experiences in the ethnic community with which she identified, she would deter other women of colour from applying to the MEP:

It's just nuts! Anybody asks how it is or ... because it's so understood like the whole world is watching the Ontario program, the rest of everywhere in the universe is watching *me*. If someone asks how the program is, it's like "Oh, it's amazing, I love it. I *never, ever* talk about ... Like I want to unload and tell [community members] how hard it is and my close friends totally know, but I don't want to give that impression because it will deter other people from applying. Like I feel like I'm the "women of colour representative," both within the program and as a midwifery student outside the program. (Interview no. 41)

Constrained to silence in the clinical setting, students of colour were often incited to speak in the classroom. In a role not unfamiliar to feminist native informants, these women found themselves helping "the First World engage in a politics of saving the women of the Third World" (Razack 2000, 42) by expanding white students' understanding of "diverse" groups. The native informant role rendered these women a reliable commodity for consumption, always available to explain, argue for, and represent undifferentiated "communities of colour." The role also accomplished an endless re-racializing of students of colour – one woman spoke of "constantly feeling like the brown chick" (Interview no. 41) – and served to absolve dominant women of the obligation to examine their own part in constructing and maintaining difference. As one student argued, "[My professor] was constantly deferring to me to talk about issues of poverty, and class and antiracist stuff. She was asking me to help teach the class. As much as on a superficial level that's kind of flattering, but then I got kind of angry, going, 'What the hell is your problem? Why aren't you struggling professionally, not just as a teacher, as professor, but as a midwife? Why aren't you working on this stuff?'" (Interview no. 43). Another woman expressed her frustration with constantly being compelled to speak in a program that propounded, as she put it, a "white liberal feminist rhetoric of [...] 'We want students who know how to work with diverse groups of people.' As opposed to 'We want a diverse group of students.' I don't want to do this. I don't want to be the educator. I don't want to be the one who talks about women of colour. And then at the same time, [I don't want to] have them not do it – not have a commitment to women of colour" (Interview no. 41).

The students were also required to perform as *authentic* native informants, who, as Sherene Razack (2000, 44) notes, are "permitted no specificities, no complexities in regard to class, histories or sexualities." One student who identified as biracial found that when she revealed her ethnicity she lost her claim to being the universal midwife. The response in the MEP, she claimed, was to assume that her mission would be to serve women of "her community." Her response was, "Like, no, I can't! I can speak their language, but I'm not accepted in their culture. When I go to [an ethnic neighbourhood] and order things and stuff, I'm a novelty; people laugh at me!" (Interview no. 42). Another woman, reflecting not on her subordination but on the privileged dimensions of her identity, remarked upon the contradiction for her of being assigned the role of authentic native informant: "I'm not the representative of Third World students! I talk white. I dress white. I was raised here. I am Canadian. I'm not an immigrant woman. Like, how much can I speak to immigrant women's needs when I'm not one? Like, I was raised in an immigrant family but when people talk about making the student body more diverse, I should not be used as an example because I'm the perfect example of the acceptable person of colour. I'm middle class" (Interview no. 41).

The three women quoted in the above section are able to "perform whiteness" by relying on class and on educational and professional knowledge that make it possible for them to participate, under conditions of daily negotiation, in the white world of midwifery. They speak unaccented English and are proficient in the languages of feminism. And, importantly, they know how to decode Canadian racism so as to protect themselves from its worst ravages. As one student put it:

> I do know that one of the reasons that I got through is that I've been raised here, and in a sense I know how to play the game. I've gone to school with these people. I've gone to school with them as a kid. And I've worked here in Canada, and so I've had to learn to cope, and part of that means being silent in certain ways, knowing when to talk and when not to. Knowing how much of yourself to ... like, in most cases, people don't know about me. They think I'm nice and quiet, they have no idea. (Interview no. 43)

The same student who refused to tell her Canadian-born racialized minority friends about her racist experiences in the MEP hurried to inform friends who were immigrant midwives of colour "not to bother" applying to the College of Midwives Prior Learning and Experience Assessment program: "I know so many people who come to me, PLEA candidates who did not get in, and now my answer is finally 'don't bother.' To have to say that to an immigrant friend of mine who's an immigrant woman from the Philippines who's trained there and has incredible skills, lives in poverty here, and to say, 'You know what, you can never get in and you won't.' Like, her writing is not middle class; you have all the skills, you speak English fine, but it's not good enough for this program" (Interview no. 41). Aware of how very difficult negotiating the white space of midwifery has been for someone like herself who possesses many of the cultural competencies linked to whiteness, this woman was perfectly positioned to see just how unlikely it was that immigrant women of colour who possessed few white cultural competencies and decoding skills would succeed in becoming registered midwives in the province of Ontario.

Midwives in Ontario have pursued a respectable identity in order to claim social parity with physicians and to make claims on the state. Among the impediments to this project is an archive of disreputable images of midwifery that has circulated for the last century and has been deployed in times of crisis to bolster the claims of modern medicine that it provides safer care to childbearing women than do traditional, unscientific practitioners. New inscriptions have been written upon the pages of these older texts and used to discredit the re-emergence of midwifery in Canada. Among the discredited figures were counterculture midwives who had been central to the reintroduction of midwifery from the 1970s onward. With the shift of the Ontario midwifery movement from a position that supported decriminalization of the practice to one that supported state funding and regulation, a new midwifery subject was required. Such a subject was unmarked by the specificities of gender and by the non-rational thought associated with "spiritual midwifery." She could make claims on the state from a liberal humanist and universal subject position. Those practising midwives who fell outside of these norms by virtue of their investments in traditional motherhood, spirituality, iconoclastic dress, and so on found themselves marginalized within the movement.

With the establishment of the Midwifery Education Program came the installation of a normative midwifery subject, "the ambassador of the profession," whose investment with white cultural competencies is highly discernible. Midwifery aspirants and students strived to produce themselves in the image of this subject, disciplining aspects of their identities that failed to align with the perceived norm. For the few students of colour admitted to the MEP, negotiating a place at the midwifery table meant maintaining a silence around difference or engaging in a form of compulsory speech that rendered them useful to midwifery's imperial project of serving diverse populations but not including them among its ranks. The normative subject at the heart of the midwifery project is one that Canadian-born or Canadian-raised women of colour who possess a significant amount of white knowledge can approximate but never fully embody. As the next chapter will demonstrate, this normative subjectivity is out of reach for most immigrant midwives of colour who have either abandoned hope of rejoining their profession in Canada or have encountered extraordinary obstacles to reclaiming a professional identity legitimately achieved in their countries of origin.

5
Narratives of Exclusion and Resistance of Women of Colour

Perpetuation of a social formation in its racialized determination is enabled both by the microexpressions which constitute it – the epithets, glances, avoidances, characterizations, prejudgements, dispositions, and rationalizations – and by the accompanying racial(izing) theories, evaluations, and behavioral recommendations. They enable, in other words, common sense to be racialized and so the easiness, the natural familiarity of racial expression.

– David Theo Goldberg, *Racist Culture*

Resistance clearly accompanies all forms of domination. However, it is not always identifiable through organized movements; resistance inheres in the very gaps, fissures, and silences of hegemonic narratives. Resistance is encoded in the practices of remembering and of writing. Agency is thus figured in the minute, day to day practices and struggles of third world women. Coherence of politics and of action comes from a sociality which itself perhaps needs to be rethought. The very practice of remembering against the grain of "public" hegemonic history, of locating the silences and the struggle to assert knowledge which is outside the parameters of the dominant suggests a rethinking of sociality itself.

– Chandra Mohanty, "Cartographies of Struggle"

Encounters between subordinate and dominant groups/individuals are never free of attachments to historical records of subjugation and discrimination (Essed 1991). Misunderstandings, breakdowns of communication, and other problematic communication events (such as those reported to me by the interview subjects) that transpire between hierarchically positioned subjects cannot, then, be viewed as mere "technical glitches" (Razack 1998b, 8). Histories of subordination must be addressed, and the trace of racial dominance must be sought in the expressions of racially privileged individuals and in the habits that structure everyday encounters with racialized minority people. To be able to recognize how our behaviours reinscribe racialized evaluations, those of us in dominant positions need to know the histories that our words and actions may perpetuate. It is in conversation that we can learn about the responses that those words and acts engender. While engaging in those conversations, we must be prepared to be accountable for how we hear what the "other" is telling us. We will never hear everything that is said, but that does not mean that we should shrink from the imperative to keep listening.

How dominantly positioned researchers work with the narratives of subordinate subjects has been the topic of much debate and little resolution. Michelle Fine and Lois Weis (1996, 266) argue that the narratives of socially privileged subjects and of those who have been "historically smothered" need to be differentially theorized and contextualized. The voices of marginalized people, they argue, should be displayed on their own terms as a form of "narrative affirmative action," whereas those of dominant group members should be subjected to "generous" theorizing, "wild" contextualizing, and "rude" interruption for the purpose of reframing. I agree with the strategy of subjecting dominant discourses to extremely rigorous treatment, and I have attempted to do so in these pages. I am less convinced, however, that "narrative affirmative action" is adequate to the task of representing the experiences of members of subordinate groups. While Fine and Weis's important work does make public narratives of poverty, racism, and violence – and I believe those efforts are laudable – I would argue that there is much to be lost by employing a strategy of simply displaying the data "performatively" (Lather 1992, 89). As Angela McRobbie (1991, 69) correctly observes, seemingly pure, uncommented-upon texts are "as ideologically loaded and as saturated with 'the subjective factor' as anything else." To under-theorize the narratives of subordinated women, then, risks having their lives equated merely with their subordinate status. Careful, respectful, and historicized contextualization and theorization of these narratives can reveal how individual encounters are embedded in larger relations of domination and subordination. Such a strategy can also interrupt the dominant subjects' rationalizations and explanations of such encounters by foregrounding subordinate group members' narrated evidence of harm. Through careful reading, it can also draw attention to forms of resistance largely invisible to racially dominant groups. And, importantly, it can endeavour to interrupt the natural relationship assumed in First World countries between a speaking subaltern subject and the culture/community/ethnic group/geographic area with which she is identified (Carr 1994). I undertake my interpretations with these possibilities in mind.

Advocating reciprocity, careful analysis, and continuous accountability in the research process can constitute yet another way that dominant subjects seek to redeem marginalized ones. What has already been demonstrated, and what should be restated here, is that power in these unequal contexts is not something that the dominant researcher necessarily confers upon subordinate research subjects. Such subjects always already exercise power in the production of research knowledge. "If one considers power as a decentralized, shifting, and productive force animated in networks of relations rather than possessed by individuals," argues Aihwa Ong (1995, 354), "then ethnographic subjects can exercise power in the production of ethnographic knowledges." Interview subjects intervene in numerous ways in the production of such forms of knowledge. The deployment of a variety of narrative strategies, such as omitting and suppressing emotion and experience, emphasizing and dramatizing the stories they offer, and euphemizing and softening what is unsayable in a direct manner, is paradigmatic of such intervention (Etter-Lewis 1993). These narratives are also crafted by the narrator in relation to the identity of the researcher, the location, and timing of the interview, the relationship established between interviewer and subject, the anticipated audience of the research, and the personal contexts that shaped the tale. I have attempted throughout this book to foreground the conditions in which all these relations of research are embedded, including legacies of imperialism, histories of transnational migration, local conditions of racial formation, and the differential impact of these conditions on women. All of these shape the subjectivities not only of those whose words are displayed, but my own as well. They shape both what I have been told and what I have heard.

In the course of this research, I interviewed three separate cohorts of women of colour and Aboriginal women. The first cohort was composed of five women who had served as representatives on midwifery boards or agencies between 1993 and 1996. Minimal demographic information is provided for these women to reduce the chance that they will be recognized, although the names of those who participated on midwifery boards and committees is a matter of public record. This cohort of women agreed to this arrangement. The second cohort was composed of immigrant midwives of colour who chose *not* to seek registration, and the third cohort represents those who *did* seek to become registered in the province through the Michener Institute program or the PLA/PLEA programs. Demographic, educational, attitudinal, and employment data for the women in cohorts two and three will be examined as a prelude to displaying and analyzing the narratives of those immigrant midwives of colour who have sought registration.

For the second and third cohorts, I offer a mapping of the following: the women's histories of migration and settlement, the scope of their education, their attitudes toward birth and medical technology, their family and class status, their work histories, and their linguistic competencies, among other demographic material. I do this not only to satisfy academic conventions but also to highlight some of the many similarities between practising midwives and those struggling to become registered. This strategy is helpful in ascertaining where boundaries between "legitimate" and "illegitimate" midwives have been drawn and in identifying the technologies that have been used to inscribe these borders.

Women of Colour and Aboriginal Women on Midwifery Boards/Bodies

> For the native, objectivity is always used against him.
>
> – Frantz Fanon, *The Wretched of the Earth*

This section explores the narratives of four women of colour and one Aboriginal woman who served on midwifery bodies between 1993 and 1996. All served formally for at least a year. To maintain some degree of anonymity for these women, I refrain from naming the boards on which they served. Nor, for anonymity's sake, do I attach any indication of ethnicity or country of origin to direct quotes from this group of women. To minimize the chance that the women's identities will be deciphered, I also make no distinction between those whose appointments were created through Orders-in-Council and those who participated voluntarily on midwifery bodies.

The number of women in this cohort is relatively small but so has been the number of women of colour represented on midwifery bodies. Those interviewed do, however, represent an appropriately broad range of racialized minority groups in the province. Of the immigrant women of colour interviewed, one woman had arrived in Canada in the mid-1970s, and the other three had been here for between ten and fifteen years at the time of the interview.[1] Three of the women came into their positions on these boards as community activists; two had no prior affiliations that linked them politically with specific communities of colour. Only three of these women were trained midwives. With the exception of Jesse Russell, a Métis woman from Thunder Bay, racialized minority women did not participate in policy-making activities related to the implementation of midwifery in Ontario until the establishment of the Transitional Council of the College of Midwives in 1993. At that time, two women of colour were appointed who had not been previously involved with midwifery in Ontario. Also in that year, an advisory council to the Prior Learning Assessment program was established on which immigrant midwives of colour served prominently, although with little impact on policies affecting women of colour who might seek registration.

Most of the women interviewed understood that they were appointed to their positions or invited to participate on boards as representatives of marginalized groups. They saw their presence as critical to the achievement of equitable access to midwifery practice for immigrant midwives of colour. Discussing her participation, one women commented, "It made me feel that midwives from other countries have a chance. I was there not for me, but because we needed to give midwives from other countries a chance" (Interview no. 8). Another woman told me, "I was really flattered that I'd been called. I did demonstrate my organizational skill and my connection with the immigrant women's group [which is what was] of interest [to the midwives]" (Interview no. 31).

Assuming that their responsibility was to speak on behalf of immigrant women of colour, some interviewees pursued that goal unself-consciously, only to be disciplined for failing to adequately represent "the public." One woman was surprised when accused, by her colleagues on a midwifery body, of lacking "objectivity" and of having a "conflict of interest" when she chose to highlight issues of particular concern to some immigrant women, most notably, the translation of midwifery promotional literature into languages other than English and French. Arguing from within the framework of midwifery discourse, she claimed that "informed choice" operated for some women only through access to language resources. She was subsequently accused of attempting to promote her community's welfare to the detriment of the "public good":

I was expected to speak out for immigrant women. I did not pussy-foot around, either; I didn't beat around the bush. Immediately, I brought up the issue of language and language barriers. I immediately asked what the plan was to overcome that. My question was: "In the past you were private practitioners, you could do whatever you like. Today, you're publicly funded. How do you overcome the language barrier to your client, not the other way around? Because they are the ones who entrusted you to meet their needs" ... Maybe they were tired of me, even in the first few meetings, bringing this up, and the answer to me was, the _____ community has to come up with their own energy to meet their needs. That was the first statement that reminded me of my place ... They said the priority was "all" women first, therefore the budget cannot be spent on one group of women. I was told I have a conflict of interest. I did always use [her native language] as an example. I don't think I'm comfortable speaking for other

ethno-racial groups. It certainly doesn't mean that they should only provide translated material [in that language]. Every time I bring up the _____
example, it is because I have a better understanding of this community.
And I was told that there's a conflict of interest there!

If it's the unique characteristic of your profession, which was not claimed
by other professions – it was not claimed by the doctors, it was not claimed
by the massage therapists – if you use that as your flag which you're waving,
communication in an appropriate language, and culturally appropriate to
get that choice understood, it's almost compulsory. It *is* compulsory. (Interview no. 31)

The questioning of this woman's ability to represent "the general public"
and the suggestion that she was acting on behalf of a "special interest group"
also arose during a meeting she chaired in which a white participant accused the College of Midwives of being biased toward immigrant women of
colour:

At one point there was a confrontation. There was a member [of a midwifery-
related body] who stood up and criticized the College of being biased toward immigrant women of colour. And when I asked her as chair, what
kind of evidence do you have, then I was shouted down by the College staff
who said that as chair, I could not challenge the person for evidence, that
this was not "facilitating" the meeting. It was done in the open. It was
totally intimidating to me as chair. And it was confusing, that meeting.

One of the Filipino representatives was upset with the member's statement and wanted to confront that person. Then I became responsible for
resolving that conflict, and the staff was not backing me up. I tried to use
my authority to ask for facts. I didn't want it to become a philosophical
debate. If the individual says the College has been biased toward immigrant
women, *not* Canadian-born women, then I want to know how and why she
said it, which is not bias, from the chair's position. I was accused by staff of
saying that I'm presenting my position which is not neutral, so I'm not
appropriate to chair that committee anymore. (Interview no. 31)

Richard Dyer (1997, 38) argues that "non-white peoples are presumed to
be still, and perhaps forever, at the stage of particular local sensations, not
having made the move to disinterested subjecthood." Caught in an impossible double bind, this woman found herself installed in a position on a midwifery board, presumably to represent marginalized women, but then was
informed that her comments and actions were tainted with self-interest.
The dominant behaviours described, without resorting to direct references
to racial inferiority, inscribe a boundary between whiteness and "otherness"

wherein white identity is ineluctably identified with "abstraction, distance, separation and objectivity"; the white person is, in Dyer's words, "everything and nothing." In this formulation, the "other" must remain mired in her particularity and is always something less than paradigmatically "woman." The "public good" can be seen as a rationalization that assumes a racializing function when deployed by dominant subjects to reassert dominance in a contested environment.

However, acquiescence to the dominant agenda, or a subsuming of interests that might be construed as particularist, did not guarantee that women of colour could participate as equals on midwifery boards. One woman of colour who truly believed that midwifery implementation was a goal that could produce gains for all women, and who even acceded to policies with which she disagreed because she believed she had to "be loyal to the College and this is what's best for all at this time" (Interview no. 8), later bemoaned her own naïveté. Included on the midwifery body in which she participated because she represented immigrant midwives of colour, she was prevented from participating directly in the formulation of policies for the Prior Learning Assessment process because, as a potential PLA participant, she was told, she had a conflict of interest.[2] Unable to use the expertise that had gained her entry to this body, she felt that her role was diminished:

> I started feeling as though my say was being dwindled and I was feeling excluded a little bit from a lot of the processes that needed to be enacted to put the PLA in place. Although I played a part in it, I still feel as though I could have played a better part, a better role. But I was isolated and I had a lot going on, too. Then I didn't think much about it because I really trusted the midwives who were on the committee to really work for us.
>
> Maybe I was a little bit naïve. Maybe I didn't know enough about government politics or the politics of a small group or a small network that was very, very strong. Maybe I was naïve to think that I would have been welcomed totally with open arms. I don't know. And that we were all going to be welcome and be a big team and playing an important role in the welfare of mothers and babies in the community. I really, really thought so. But looking back now, I thought I was a bit naïve, thinking that it was going to work well. (Interview no. 8)

Her subsequent comments demonstrate how the "heroic tale" of midwifery's struggle for recognition was used to defer claims of inequity:

> Years later, the process is not working and I can't see it working until changes are made and the attitudes of practising midwives right now change. Because they're still on a high and they still have this feeling that they are

invincible, you know: "They can wait, foreign-trained midwives can wait because we've waited so long to get where we are today, they can wait a bit longer." (Interview no. 8)

New to Canada and to the politics of midwifery in Ontario, this woman could not fully anticipate the obstacles or adequately decode the exclusionary moves that would impede her participation as a midwife of equal stature on the board on which she served. Being the only immigrant midwife of colour on this particular body made expressing opposition difficult. It is striking that for neither of the women quoted is a viable subject position available. For the first woman, active advocacy on behalf of communities of colour – the stance she willingly assumes on the board – is branded as "not acting in the public interest." For the second woman, attempts to claim the unmarked subject position of "midwife" are thwarted when her foreign training and outsider status are seen to constitute a "conflict of interest" in participating on the PLA/PLEA process. Whether they claimed identities that asserted or subsumed their status as racialized minority women, the women were marked as incapable of objectivity. Within the midwifery movement, those who made special claims needed to be contained so that the illusion of a "public good" could be maintained and so that exclusions could be narrated as justifiable. Those who expressed loyalties or demonstrated ties to specific groups appear to have been construed as inadequate to the task of formulating "public" policy.

As Philomena Essed (1991, 147) has remarked, racialized minority women's comprehension of racism is not a function of "common sense" but is acquired, rather, through a "deliberate problematization of social reality." Two non-midwife participants in midwifery boards, women who had lived in Ontario for more than twenty years and who had years of community activism behind them, drew on sophisticated analyses and prior experiences of exclusion to construct their narratives of participation. One woman offered a complex criticism, drawn from a history of past struggles, of the tokenism that had characterized her role on one midwifery board. As a woman of colour who did not display deference to the white board members with whom she served, she was often left out of the information loop, a practice which, as Leroy Wells (1998, 396) has noted, "has the effect of disempowering, disenfranchising, and marginalizing" racialized minority people in white-dominated work settings. "Moreover," argues Wells, "the combination of ambiguous communication, unreliable information, and incomplete feedback creates an unstable and highly stressful work environment with significant negative effects on the role occupant." While occupying a position of putative power, this woman felt that informal forces undermined her ability to deploy such power. Her description of her role as chair of a committee demonstrates that covert manoeuvres of influence are difficult for isolated and racialized people to challenge, and that larger circuits of racialized power always structure relations at the micro level:

> I only managed to chair that committee for a year, that's when I played a leadership role. And that was very interesting. Decisions were made behind my back, undermining my position as a leader. There was also a veto; it was not my decision, it was the committee's decision by a more informal powerful clique. Even in the [recorded] minutes, a decision was made that two days later was changed because the more influential members of the movement decided that it isn't what they want. I asked why that was and basically I was told, "Oh, we just want to get the work done fast. Oh, you weren't consulted? Oh, it's not intentional." But the undercurrent statement is "What can you do about it?" I think part of this is so-called racist practice ... I'm seeing a pattern that intimidation is a challenge, so you have no clout, so you have the foremost position to do certain things but you can't do it. The system is not on your side, the social system we're talking about. So who are you going to complain to? So what are you going to do about it? (Interview no. 31)

Like the woman who participated in Interview no. 8, this woman referred to her sense of isolation on the midwifery body. Early in our conversation, she had negotiated the terms of her interview. Caution needed to be taken, she told me, because she was one of the few women of colour who had served on a midwifery board and one of the few who does a particular kind of advocacy work for women of colour. The lack of a critical mass of women like herself made it dangerous for her to speak out without jeopardizing future projects. "I don't have a collectivity" she told me. "If there is a collective, the anonymity is not as relevant" (Interview no. 31). Recognizing that isolation is an inevitable companion to tokenism, and having served as a "token" woman of colour innumerable times, she evaluated how that role was constructed for her on a midwifery body:

> Yes, a token, well, I mean, realistically let's face it ... in the process of inclusiveness, you couldn't possibly invite people of colour other than [as] tokens. Meaning that you couldn't even invite a representative percentage of people to sit on [a midwifery body]. I'm not that euphoric to believe that. The fact that they recognize [her advocacy work] ... is an improvement. So the entry point is pretty innocent. But when it comes to crisis time, like decision making, like the distribution of resources, those are the issues, and also like why is a decision made behind my back? So there is lack of full disclosure. (Interview no. 31)

In the wake of her problematic participation on a midwifery body, this woman articulated so clearly the conditions for "full partnership," whereby women otherwise hierarchically positioned might actually participate and benefit equally from a shared project. She suggested that accountability to a more broadly and diversely conceptualized public requires that power be shared:

> So what my experience is, therefore, I learned ... in genuine partnership there are three F's. The first one is full disclosure, the second one is full participation ... And the third thing is full sharing of resources. I learned that. Those are the criteria for genuine partnership. So I'm not saying that when you and I meet together you have to address me by my [non-Anglicized] name, I'm not demanding that. I'm rather looking to these three aspects to make it meaningful: full disclosure, full participation, and full sharing of the resources on this project. I don't want to share your house, but when you're doing that work to bring this common goal, the common goal is to make this service available to the public so, because this is a publicly funded profession now and the public would feel it's worthwhile to fund this project. (Interview no. 31)

This interviewee also elucidated the material conditions that constrained the participation of women of colour and Aboriginal women on voluntary and appointed midwifery bodies. Access to flexible employment, Western academic and (white) cultural competencies, and generous domestic support systems are fundamental conditions for participating in what this woman calls "governance work." Some of these resources are in short supply for immigrant women of colour and Aboriginal women. The material conditions described are unavailable to some immigrant midwives of colour, whose educational qualifications may have been gained outside of Canada, whose employment conditions (for example, in nursing or home-based health or child care) may have been rigidly controlled, and whose access to extended family or community supports may have been limited owing to geographic dislocation. In outlining the conditions under which "full participation" she can be achieved, she outlined how involvement in public projects works differently for women who are positioned subordinately in the social matrix:

> I hope people realize that for an immigrant woman to participate in this kind of governance work, which has irregular hours, irregular demands, expectations, you need the kind of resource ... the kind of job that you can go in and out of freely and the kind of family life you can go in and out of to produce that ... Because a lot of them would say, "Oh, its not that we don't want to include women of colour: it's just that there aren't too many of them who have that kind of skill." I can't accept that, you know. I'm

talking about social resources. I'm talking about I could be a professor from [a country in the South], and yet I don't have the kind of job which allows me to go in and out and come to your meetings.[3] I don't have the kind of family support system that I can push aside my child care and come to, to produce that kind of work ...

At one point, Aboriginal women were criticized – "She can't head a certain committee because she can't present briefs" – and I contradicted that to say, "If writing skills are what you want, you can easily contract a university student to do that. But you are talking about these Aboriginal women who have rich knowledge and experience within the Aboriginal midwifery service.[4] That's what you want, her ideas, not her writing skill. You can contract a student to sit side by side with her, get that idea out." That suggestion was pushed aside. (Interview no. 31)

Another woman, a long-time advocate for immigrant women of colour, harboured few expectations about the impact of her presence on the midwifery body on which she served. Her unenthusiastic description of the meetings that she had attended attested to how the participation and input of women of colour was regulated. "They were friendly meetings. They allowed us to express ourselves, of course. It was not bad, basically, let's put it that way" (Interview no. 30). The frustration that she felt in not seeing immigrant midwives of colour gain a foothold in midwifery in Ontario was no different, she explained, than what she had experienced in the other campaigns for employment equity, where the threat of lower professional standards always arose when immigrant people of colour sought inclusion. When asked if she felt that she had influenced policy, she responded:

No, I don't think so, but I wanted more to do because I know it's difficult to influence policy unless you're inside, right? And unless you know the steps to go about it. But ... my goal wasn't for them [the midwifery movement]. What I wanted to say was, "There are qualified midwives here; what they need is a chance to just prove themselves" ... The frustration is just like in all groups when you try to push for accreditation. They think that if they include people from Third World countries ... that they are lowering their standards. They are not, they're just opening up the pool, right? So I guess that's the frustration, it seems like they keep on harping on "standards, standards" but basically we're not saying "lower the standards"; we're just saying "open it up." (Interview no. 30)

Four out of five of the representatives interviewed felt that they had been marginalized during their participation on a midwifery body, and at least one woman believed that she had also failed the people she supposedly represented. Having spent considerable time consulting with groups of

immigrant midwives of colour that had begun to meet informally in antici-
pation of the Prior Learning Assessment initiative, this woman felt that
despite her own best efforts she had not managed to influence policies that
would speed their entrance to midwifery practice:

> Through networking into the community – because I believe that commu-
> nity is important, because it is the community that midwives will be serv-
> ing – we met with the Filipino Midwives Association, the Chinese [Canadian
> Nurses] Association, I got in contact with a couple of women I knew mi-
> grated and met occasionally here. They're spread all over the place and I
> contacted them and networked with some other midwives who are nurse-
> midwives from home and encouraged them, "Let's get together." Some came
> to my home and I said, "Let me update you with what we're doing," and
> they were quite thrilled. They could see me playing that role and ... they
> wanted a part in the process.
>
> When they saw that they had a nurse-midwife from this country, they
> were quite thrilled and they contacted the College and they wanted to meet
> us. And they asked me to speak at a couple of their ... they wanted my
> background and they wanted ... they got that contact that they had some-
> body there for them. And I started feeling really, really like I had this whole
> weight, all these women on my shoulders and I felt so disappointed by the
> time proclamation had taken place, I kept saying, "Oh, my God, there is no
> way. We're not going to have midwives from other countries starting to
> practise, not maybe for the next ten years or so" ... There's a lot of things
> being said in ... outside, here, in the community, that you're not sure you
> should say you were involved at all. But I say it anyway. Because with a clear
> conscience, I can say that I tried and I really worked hard with my limited
> whatever, if they think it was limited knowledge or whatever it is. But I
> thought I brought a lot of experience and I was able to bring a lot to the
> College. (Interview no. 8)

Constrained and circumvented by covert circuits of power and locked
into an untenable role as the "other" whose contribution is never construed
as objective or as linked to the "public good," the women of colour whom I
interviewed who participated on midwifery boards just prior to and for the
three years following proclamation of midwifery legislation felt that, despite their considerable investment of time and energy, they had not succeeded in opening up midwifery practice to immigrant women of colour.

Immigrant Midwives of Colour Who Did Not Seek Registration
Five immigrant midwives of colour who chose not to pursue registration
were interviewed in the course of this research. Hundreds of foreign-trained
midwives attended midwifery information meetings just following legal-

ization, but relatively few ultimately pursued registration. I conducted interviews with this group to determine why some immigrant midwives of colour decided against participating in the PLA/PLEA process. Their comments and the accompanying demographic information suggest possible explanations rather than verifiable trends among these women.

Four of the women interviewed had immigrated to Canada in the mid-1980s and one had come in 1994. Like many people of colour in Ontario, four of these women lived in suburban areas and commuted into an urban area to work. One woman both lived and worked within an urban area. All were currently in their late thirties or early forties. Two of the five women had followed the multi-stop immigration routes so common in the transnational flow of immigrants, including one well known to Filipino nurses: Philippines, Saudia Arabia, Canada (Stasiulis and Bakan 2003, 123; Joyce and Hunt 1982) and one familiar to Afro-Caribbean women (particularly nurses, who often pursue basic or advanced training in the UK): Caribbean country, England, Canada (Rashid 1990). Four of these women held nursing positions at the time of the interview, including (sometimes simultaneously because of part-time staffing) as public health nurses and nurse practitioners, and as labour and delivery nurses. The woman who had most recently immigrated worked as a home care worker and as an occasional second attendant in a midwifery practice. One of the women had entered Canada as a live-in caregiver even though she had full credentials as a nurse and midwife at the time.

All five of the women interviewed had completed three years of post-secondary nursing training and between one and two years of specialized midwifery education. All had been trained in prenatal care, although this is not necessarily a part of midwifery training in some countries. Many in the Ontario midwifery community perceived foreign-trained midwives to be opposed to home birth. However, this cohort, as well as an overwhelming majority of the cohort of PLA/PLEA participants interviewed for this study, expressed no such opposition and had been trained to attend home births in their countries of origin.

While there are numerous possible reasons why immigrant midwives of colour might not have sought registration, for some the stringency of the registration requirements denigrated their hard-won skills and credentials. For one woman who had undergone three years of nursing training and two years of speciality midwifery training, not participating in the PLA/PLEA process was a way of reasserting her rightful status as a midwife: "For me, I think that I have my midwife licence and I don't need people to evaluate me. That's what that is! [laughter]. I think I'm competent enough to work in the midwife role, but in case they have to assess me again and have me do everything, I say that's just too much time and involvement, so I'd better not" (Interview no. 5).

In the same vein, another woman declared, "I'm not sure I even want to practise; I just want recognition for my credential" (Interview no. 29). Denigration of skills was also raised in relation to the profession-specific language exam. One woman for whom English was a second language acceded to the need for English testing for those for whom English was not their first language, but reported the negative responses of her co-workers, many of whom were trained in England, to the requirement for an English examination:[5] "They said, 'Why do they [native English speakers trained in the UK] have to take the English exam? You know, their first language is English. For us, that is not our first language so even if it is mandatory, it is okay for us.' But for the American and British nurses, they said that if they will exclude the exam, then many nurses from England will do [the PLEA process]" (Interview no. 2).

One of the likely reasons that some women did not choose to pursue registration was that they had, for some time, been working in stable and relatively well-paying nursing jobs. Pursuing registration would have meant losing income, owing to the time required to study and to attend mandatory courses. One woman spoke of valuing stability, an arguably precious commodity for those whose lives have been punctuated by transnational migrations: "My job is stable and secure and I prefer to just be in that role, not look for any particular change" (Interview no. 5). Another woman referred to the extensive demands on the time and resources of those pursuing registration; "Some of us have to work for a living," she said (Interview no. 29). For these women, cost was also identified as a significant deterrent to seeking registration through the PLA/PLEA program.

Two of those interviewed worked in an urban hospital that was noted for serving a racially and ethnically diverse population as well as for the high percentage of foreign-trained midwives, largely women of colour, who worked in its labour and delivery department. For this unique group, lack of interest in pursuing regulation may be related to the fact that, in this workplace, midwives working as labour and delivery nurses received a significant amount of recognition from both doctors and families for their midwifery skills. While rarely able to provide the continuity of perinatal care that is a cornerstone of the midwifery model and for which some were trained, these women were able to perform a range of tasks roughly equivalent, in some cases, to those they had performed when working as midwives in their countries of origin or of training, including conducting the actual delivery of the baby, a task usually performed exclusively by physicians. Reported one woman, "We are checking the patient, examining the patient, delivering the patient, especially when the doctor cannot make it" (Interview no. 5). Another woman working in this hospital said, "We do deliver the babies with the doctor's signature; that means the doctor has to check everything to make sure of everything. Our doctors are supposed to be in there twenty-four hours, but they are not. They are not. We [nurses] often are the prime person to look after everything" (Interview no. 2).

Asked whether she felt that her own experience as an immigrant was part of the expertise that she offered her patients, this woman described how well-respected she felt by the largely immigrant population she served. She contrasted the trust shown her by patients in this hospital with the questioning of her authority that occurs in a suburban hospital in which she also works:

> I think that because of the relationship with the nurses and, you know, the family, and so on, because if they see kind of the same language, same-looking, you come from the same places, they trust you. And then they more rely on you. If the doctor is not here, sometimes that's fine because "Mrs. ____" – they usually call you by the last name because it's a show of respect – "as long as you're here, it's okay. If you think that it is good, go ahead and do so." [...] There's more trust and [the patients] allow us to do a little bit more, I think [...] They don't all the time say, "I want to speak to the doctor" and "Can I speak to the doctor first". (Interview no. 2)

The opportunities for communication and mutual respect this woman describes may or may not be related to the unique environment in which she works, where a largely racialized minority patient population, many of whom had emigrated from countries where midwifery care was the norm, was likely to encounter an immigrant midwife of colour during labour and delivery. The sense of authority conveyed by these women (and by several others whom I encountered in the Humber College/Women's College Hospital childbirth educators program), together with their relative lack of interest in pursuing midwifery registration, raises numerous questions about the dynamics of subordination and dominance in a space in which caregivers of colour were present in significant numbers. In the absence of any substantive data about such dynamics, I can only conjecture that immigrant midwives of colour working as nurses in such a space might have preferred to remain in an environment where they expected and received a degree of respect not accorded them in white-dominated spaces. One of the women interviewed, who was clearly cognizant that midwifery in Ontario was dominated by white midwives and white clients, commented, "The thing is, you know, all the midwifery clients are Caucasian, eh?; they're white. So maybe they don't really need those coloured people to help them to deliver" (Interview no. 2).

Some of the women also expressed a fear of increased vulnerability if they were to work with midwifery's largely white clientele. Three expressed fear of being held legally liable in the event of charges of malpractice, were they to become registered midwives. Some had already encountered several litigious patients. One woman observed that in her experience "non-immigrant" patients were more likely to sue caregivers of colour than were immigrant patients of colour: "Yeah, I don't know why they are doing that. That is, according to my observation, those non-immigrants they will just come here to deliver their babies, then complicated ... something's wrong with the baby or sometimes something is wrong with them and then they will blame the hospital, the doctors, and the nurses" (Interview no. 5).

There is, I believe, a complex set of impulses that leads immigrant women of colour to fear the threat of lawsuits. Perhaps the ability to practise midwifery is not worth the risk of a serious challenge to their professional credibility, stability, and material resources. As Frantz Fanon (1992, 225) reminds us, "The black physician can never be sure how close he is to disgrace." The person of colour invested with professional expertise always seems anomalous in white society and her/his expertise is constantly under the threat of erasure.

Unlike the other women interviewed, who as hospital labour and delivery nurses had received numerous notices about routes to registration in the years prior to legalization, the most recent immigrant among this cohort, a home-based child care worker, had not applied to the PLEA program because she did not know it existed. I contacted this woman through a midwifery practice where she was working occasionally as a second attendant.[6] Because I knew that two members of this practice had recently completed the PLEA, I was taken aback to learn that this woman had not been encouraged by her colleagues to pursue registration. One veteran midwife at the practice expressed a sense of being besieged by too many women of colour and was unable to imagine taking on a second woman from a specific racialized minority group because she already used a second attendant from that group "at these births." (The woman I interviewed was that attendant.) The failure of the midwives with whom she worked to inform her about and encourage her to seek registration is a prime example of how racist exclusion can be effected through passive practices. A midwife with more than twenty years of experience from her country of origin, this woman was excited to learn about the prospect of becoming registered and I subsequently mailed her a copy of the CMO's PLEA booklet.

Immigrant Midwives of Colour:
Microprocesses of Exclusion and the Pursuit of Registration
Between July 1996 and November 1998, I interviewed twelve immigrant midwives of colour who had pursued registration. Only two of the women were registered and practising at the time of the interview. Of the twelve,

two had participated in the Michener Institute Pre-registration Program, three had participated in the first cycle of the PLA/PLEA process, which began in October 1994, and seven participated in cycle two, which began in October 1997. This breakdown is significant because cycle one of the PLEA is recognized by officials of the College of Midwives as having been significantly more problematic than cycle two. In an interview conducted in March of 1998, CMO Registrar Robin Kilpatrick described the first cycle:

> But I think in terms of cycle one, we've come to see it as a prototype, meaning that you just try it out. You know it's not the model that you're going to end up with. You know it's not the best. It's the working model to see where's the problems ...
>
> So there were extremely long delays in the process that obviously affected the individual candidates' confidence. This concerns all sorts of things that were part of going through a process that was in development ... And certainly cycle one was painful in some ways for everyone, including the College. (Interview with CMO Registrar Robin Kilpatrick and PLEA Coordinator Jill Moriarity, 11 March 1998)

Cycle one participants experienced more bureaucratic errors and delays, and such errors and delays are frequently interpreted by women of colour as racism in light of their personal experience or of their knowledge of exclusionary behaviours toward people of colour. Cycle two participants, however, reported that the bureaucratic streamlining of the PLA/PLEA process did not diminish racially defined experiences. It might be argued that an equal number of participants from cycle one and cycle two would have given a more balanced picture of the PLA/PLEA process, but the predominance of cycle two participants allows an analysis of racially defined incidents that are presumably less intertwined with bureaucratic incompetence and theoretically are more transparent to interpretation.[7]

Participants came from all the global regions from which Ontario has received immigrants in the last twenty years. Four women were born in the Caribbean. Three identified their origins as Afro-Caribbean, one as Indo-Caribbean. Two had emigrated from Africa, and one had come from the Philippines. Three had immigrated to Ontario from East or Southeast Asia. One woman had emigrated from an Arab country and one had come from Central America. For eight of the twelve women interviewed, Canada was the second, third, or even fourth country they had migrated to after leaving their countries of birth. For most, having come from British Commonwealth nations in the South, England was the first port in their transnational migration, although Saudi Arabia and the United States had been stops for two of the women.

Of the twelve, seven were native English speakers and five spoke English as a second language, although one had resided and worked for twenty years in an English-speaking country.[8] Participants ranged in age from mid-twenties to late fifties with an estimated average age of forty-three. The women had immigrated to Canada between 1981 and 1996. Half had arrived within the five years previous to the interview. Seven were working as nurses, two were working as midwives, and two worked in midwifery-related or childbirth-related jobs at the time of the interview. One woman, who possessed a four-year bachelor's degree in midwifery from her country of origin, was employed as a telemarketer, and one worked as a home health-care aide. Nine out of the twelve women described middle-class upbringings in their countries of origin, with parents who were teachers, physicians, or business owners. The remaining three were raised in working-class homes.

With one exception, all the immigrant midwives of colour interviewed had obtained nursing and midwifery credentials in government-accredited schools. All – with the exception of one woman who had simultaneously earned a bachelor's degree in history and midwifery – had completed three-year registered nursing studies programs and had earned a midwifery credential during additional studies lasting from one to two years. Before emigrating, one woman had been sent by government health officials to receive special training in the United States, in family planning techniques and advanced midwifery. Another had pursued an additional year of training as a public health nurse after completing her nursing and midwifery credentials.

Those women who had undergone nursing training in their countries of origin and had arrived in the ten years prior to the interview had little difficulty passing the nursing entrance exams or gaining equivalency from the College of Nurses of Ontario to become licensed, and most entered nursing careers immediately upon arrival in Canada. However, one woman who arrived in the early 1980s from a Southeast Asian country was compelled to repeat her RN degree to be able to practise in Ontario. Only one woman was an empirically trained midwife who had studied not in her country of origin but in the United States as an apprentice midwife. Half of the women had completed their education in Great Britain.

This group, perhaps more than any of the others, exercised considerable power in the research encounter. On two occasions women seized the agenda before I had a chance to begin the interview. Arriving at one of my first interviews with an immigrant midwife of colour, I found her waiting with a list of questions related to her upcoming PLEA exam. As I will argue, access to knowledge related to midwifery in Ontario was not easily obtained by immigrant midwives of colour, and the woman at this interview availed herself of a rare opportunity to get direct answers to her questions. We worked our way systematically through her questions before beginning the interview process. At a different interview, I became the object of a surprising reversal when the interview subject began to interrogate me about why I, as a white women, would be so interested in issues affecting women of colour.

Immigrant Midwives of Colour and Midwifery Philosophies

Eleven out of the twelve women interviewed indicated that they largely embraced the same philosophical tenets as Ontario-trained midwives. The fear among some midwifery supporters that foreign-trained midwives held a "different philosophy of continuity of care, choice of birthplace, and informed choice" (Matthews and Thatcher 1992, 21) appears unfounded in light of the interviews I conducted. Eleven of the women described their experience with home births. While these ranged from attendance at only a handful of home births to "hundreds and hundreds" (Interview no. 8), all eleven women considered themselves competent and willing to attend women who chose to give birth at home. One immigrant midwife of colour, cognizant of Ontario midwifery philosophy as well as of the claim that foreign-trained midwives, particularly those who had emigrated from Britain, had an overly medical approach to childbirth, refuted such a charge by claiming, emphatically, to be better prepared to attend home births than women trained in Ontario:

> In my training I was taught to give people ... to make sure that the clients have informed choice and I know what that means and I know how to do that. Choice of birth place: most of the births that I have done have been in hospitals but I know that if a client wanted a home birth I feel confident to do that because the setting that I've worked in has equipped me to deal with emergencies. Whereas I know that some of the midwives here that trained in Toronto that have been practising prior to legislation haven't come across some of the emergencies that I've come across, haven't had to deal with some of the emergencies that I've had to deal with in a legitimate way, obviously because they couldn't take on high-risk clients, for starters. They weren't allowed to deal with obstetrical emergencies. They weren't allowed to assist with obstetrical emergencies. Once things became complicated they had to hand the case over. Whereas midwives trained in England have to follow through. (Interview no. 7)

Claims that foreign-trained midwives were enamoured of medicalized childbirth sometimes carry a pejorative subtext in which Third World medical systems are viewed as the outdated remnants of British imperialism. Third World people appear in this formulation to slip from the mooring of their ontological positioning as "traditional" and "non-technological" by mimicking the ill-advised obsession with technology that has infected the West. However, the women interviewed frequently resisted such claims and their inferiorizing subtexts, even asserting that the systems of maternity care from which they had come were superior to those encountered in Canada. One woman who had served on a midwifery board, and who was familiar with midwifery ideologies that eschewed unnecessary technology and championed women's choice, used that discourse to argue that, unlike in Canada, maternity care in her country of origin had never employed coercive, inhumane, nor inefficacious forms of care. Her narrative offers a vigorous resistance to claims that foreign-trained midwives were ideologically opposed to the philosophy of care in Ontario:

> To be honest, I find that the system that we use at home, because we have this one-on-one, this on-touch, this is not a lot of technology interfering. I find it a superior system ... I look at it from this angle: we don't have people being hooked up and strapped down with machines to check baby heart rate, fetal monitor, and all the time these women can't walk around as they want. *We* don't do that! *We* give women the opportunity to walk as they want, do what they want during labour. The freedom to move. *We* don't tell them they have to be strapped up like this and lie flat on their back if they don't want to ...
>
> I had to fight to observe three Caesareans when I was doing midwifery back home. If the same course was here, I would have to fight to see a normal delivery without an episiotomy.[9] In all my years that I have been a midwife, I did one episiotomy and that was because I was delivering a preterm infant ... I thought I was coming to this industrialized country with everything in place and I was going to move on. I never thought that I was going to be at the bottom of the barrel and struggling to be recognized for what I am and for what I have done, for who I am. (Interview no. 8)

Six of the twelve women interviewed had received their training in Great Britain, and two had completed this training within five years of the date that the interview was conducted. Their views indicate that, contrary to fears that British-trained midwives were more comfortable with a subordinate and medically oriented role in childbirth, recent midwifery graduates from the UK were philosophically in agreement with the principles of Ontario midwifery. While there had been a decline in the 1970s of British midwives' autonomy, which was linked to the decrease in the number of home births in England, various forces arose to challenge medicalized childbirth and the diminution of the midwife's role (Isherwood 1995). Consequently, recent graduates were trained in an atmosphere in which challenges to medical dominance in childbirth were familiar, and those interviewed expressed maternity-care politics congruent with the critical views of such groups as England's Association of Radical Midwives (Weitz 1987), which are similar to those espoused by Ontario midwives. One such woman, who has had extended experience with an Ontario midwifery practice, declared the Ontario system to be "a carbon copy of our philosophy, our training, and our system" (Interview no. 7). However, the PLA/PLEA process appears not to have been identical for white British-trained midwives and their racialized minority counterparts. I will return to this point.

Half of those interviewed had some basic knowledge about the way midwifery was practised in Ontario before they began the Michener Institute Pre-registration Program or the PLA/PLEA process. Three had been enrolled in the Humber College/Women's College Hospital childbirth educators program, where the curriculum included substantial material on Ontario midwifery and childbirth reform. One had learned about Ontario's system from her colleagues in the Association of Radical Midwives in England, who considered it "the ideal model of midwifery" (Interview no. 1). Another woman had actually worked as a midwife prior to legislation and one woman had been working as a second attendant in a midwifery practice since coming to Ontario. However, only intimate knowledge of midwifery practice and the culture of alternative birth – resources available largely to white women – offered any advantage in the struggle to become registered.

One woman disagreed with many aspects of Ontario midwifery practice. She regarded home birth as unsafe (but was prepared, nonetheless, to conduct births at home) and felt it wise to defer to medical authority in most matters related to childbirth. She also expressed distaste for the emphasis on sexuality in some of the assessments she had undergone, which tested the extent of her knowledge on accommodating diversity in childbearing. She was particularly distressed by the requirement to understand the contexts and particular needs of lesbian women and their families. However, among the seventeen immigrant midwives of colour interviewed, her views are entirely singular. They are antithetical to the views on midwifery practice expressed by every other woman interviewed. A remarkable confluence exists between the professional knowledge and philosophical bent of the midwives interviewed for this study and the scope of practice and philosophy of care of registered midwives in Ontario. In addition, the majority of those interviewed had worked in the health care system in Ontario, spoke English fluently or relatively fluently, and had some knowledge of the policies and practices of Ontario midwives. Despite these confluences, many of those interviewed found that routines of racism and forms of exclusion awaited them as they navigated the long and arduous road to registration. Of the ten women interviewed who had participated in the PLA/PLEA program, only two became eligible for registration and only one is currently practising.

"White Knowledge": Unequal Access to Midwifery Resources

In February 1998, I attended a meeting of the Toronto Association of Aspiring Midwives (TAAM). Established several years before by women hoping to gain entrance to the Midwifery Education Program, the group identifies itself in its promotional flyer as "a collective of women committed to grassroots organizing and community education who are of the belief that pregnancy and childbirth are healthy, physiological, emotional, spiritual and transformative life events." It also functions as "a support network and study group which relies on the sharing of our individual knowledge skills, and training, [drawing] on outside resources [texts, videos, etc.] and other individuals' expertise." Of the nine women attending the meeting, eight were working as doulas: women trained to provide emotional and physical support (but no clinical services) for labouring women and their families. One woman was also a student midwife. All were white. In the course of the last few years, more than half of the group's members have been admitted to the Midwifery Education Program. In a program that accepts only one out of every fifteen applicants, this is an impressive achievement.

What struck me as I sat in the meeting was the extraordinary access these women had to the resources that could pave their way into the profession by making them desirable candidates for the Midwifery Education Program. These resources provided precisely the kinds of knowledge many immigrant midwives of colour lacked. I recalled, for example, the stack of outdated public library books on home birth and North American midwifery that one midwife of colour had on her table during our interview. That collection represented the extent of her access to a complex culture of alternative birth in which a variety of esoteric knowledge and cultural competencies held sway. Over my nineteen years of childbirth reform activism, my own shelves had grown crowded with obscure and expensive journals, books obtained from specialized stores and catalogues, and films, pamphlets, and other material acquired from years of attending conferences both in and outside of North America. Unlike the woman I had interviewed, TAAM members had found numerous avenues through which to access this body of knowledge. Many participated in a variety of volunteer activities that put them in contact with midwives, doulas, childbirth educators, and others who provided access to information about birthing alternatives. The presence in this group of university-educated women who had graduated from Women's Studies programs guaranteed that feminist formulations, understood to be the lingua franca of the Midwifery Education Program, framed discussions of reproductive health and care and allowed TAAM members to absorb and process some of the vocabulary of feminism to which they might not otherwise be exposed. And, once TAAM members began to be accepted into the MEP, intimate knowledge of the attributes of the normative midwifery subject became increasingly available. One TAAM member described to me all that she had done to maximize her chances of acceptance:

> I did palliative care on a volunteer basis with people with AIDS and I did the same work for pay, low pay, in a home care agency. I did a lot of volunteer work with teens who are mostly single having babies in the hospital with doctors who didn't have any support. So I became the labour support. I did do a training, I attended midwifery conferences in the United States. Like I knew what I had to do and I took advantage of the access and resources ... I didn't know anyone until I did that TAAM thing and started volunteering ... And suddenly, I, very quickly, almost overnight, like had it all at my fingertips! I was, like, at the centre of it all, you know? Where I went and what I did and how I got there, and all because of my background and my university training and, I think, a degree in Women's Studies in terms of just knowing how to just ... I think ... something like knowing the lingo of feminism or feminisms to, you know, make things work. (Interview no. 35)

Another TAAM member who later became a midwifery student told me, "I talked to all of them [TAAM members] and I met with some of them and I tried to figure out, I didn't know where you volunteer, where you go to get experience, who do you talk to, what are the organizations? And all these people were involved, they had knowledge" (Interview no. 36).

I identify this corpus of information as "white knowledge," knowledge available largely within and through networks of white women whose lives intersect only minimally with those of women of colour. Women of colour struggled for access to these forms of knowledge, not always successfully, and their absence from an otherwise sound repertoire of midwifery competencies affected these women's abilities to successfully negotiate assessments and a variety of other interactions with white midwives and with the Ontario midwifery bureaucracy.

Lack of familiarity with midwifery practice in Ontario constituted one of the key information deficits for the women interviewed. One immigrant midwife of colour who had nearly completed the PLEA program at the time of the interview complained that "there was no real guidance for those who went through it first of all, so all those who didn't have a good understanding of how things work in Ontario were at a disadvantage from the word go. And that when it came to the sort of the periphery of midwifery, not the actual core skills, many of us were foundering, finding ways of getting a good grounding so that we could move on" (Interview no. 15).

Although an education module on practice issues was included as part of the Prior Learning and Experience Assessment process, it was one of the last components of the program. Most of the non-practising immigrant mid-wives of colour whom I interviewed had never visited a midwifery practice in Ontario. Some who had attempted to gain local knowledge of midwifery through contact with practising midwives had encountered obstacles, oc-casionally in the form of everyday racist practices. A woman who came close to finishing but ultimately dropped out of the PLEA program spoke about how, after seeking out a midwifery practice where she might learn about the local realities, she was relegated to housekeeping work rather than . treated as a colleague:

> I talked to the [midwifery practice] group and asked if it was possible some-time during the week, if I'm not working, to come in and observe how they do their practice. And she said yes, so that day I went in. She sent me into the storage room while she put up the charts and did all the paperwork. And then when a client came, she didn't want me to be there ... you need the client's agreement. She said, "I'll call you later and see which client I can get to agree," but never, never. (Interview no. 3)

A woman who had served on a midwifery board and was herself a mid-wife described her efforts to link Ontario midwives with foreign-trained midwives in the period just following implementation of the legislation. Regarded with suspicion by those she approached, and reduced, despite her position on a midwifery board, to supplicant status, she nonetheless framed her narrative as a story about how to establish professional parity between Ontario midwives and those trained elsewhere:

> Let's get midwives or women to work with these other [immigrant] mid-wives to share their experiences together, to work as a unit. Let us do it. They're begging. I begged. I begged, I had to really beg! I don't know what else to say, I went on my knees and I begged "please," but it wasn't met with openness. It wasn't an open ... it took a little begging. I was in negotiation, I literally begged to see what they did. And it wasn't because I wanted to monitor them. It wasn't like that. It was to share the same love, the same experience. And they could have done the same. (Interview no. 8)

A woman who had been my student in the Humber College/Women's College Hospital childbirth educators program, and who had abandoned the PLEA process after waiting a year for a response to her application, which she subsequently discovered had been lost by the College of Midwives, com-mented on how her pursuit of registration might have gone differently if she had had access to more knowledge about the way the midwifery appa-ratus functioned. "I was excited," she recalled, "and I was new and there was nobody to guide me, like someone inside from ... like a midwife or maybe if I'd met you at the time, it would have been different! But I didn't know anybody from inside there or someone who could tell me that you have to be careful" (Interview no. 9).

Another example of a "white knowledge" requirement for immigrant midwives of colour was that they be able to interpret and translate cultural difference attributed to a variety of cultural "others." In the example below, a recently arrived woman who had received high marks on her clinical examinations talked about one examination she had failed:

> Interviewee no. 15: There were questions that I remember saying to some of the others in the group that [the test] was asking about Native Indians and this particular couple wanted to burn blue grass or some kind of grass.
>
> Sheryl: Sweet grass?
>
> Interviewee no. 15: Sweet grass, as part of the cultural, you know, around birth and the fire regulations in the hospital were such that the smoke detector – how would you sort of work it so that the couple were, their needs were taken into consideration plus the hospital's? I had no – I mean I'd read about culture but that wasn't one of the things that I thought I'd answered very well. I wasn't so sure about what the meanings were for the couple of the blue grass or in fact what blue grass is and how broad that could be so ... I suggested burning it outside the window, somewhere outside and that was one that I just hadn't answered very well ... I don't have any problems with anything to do specifically with midwifery. It's mainly with the issues that might be mainly the Ontario way of doing things. (Interview no. 15)

There are several troubling aspects to the requirement that immigrant midwives of colour display mastery of decontextualized fragments of cultural knowledge for various marginalized groups in Ontario. For recent immigrants, practical knowledge of how differently positioned minoritized groups negotiate medical care in the province cannot be acquired organically within a short time, and acquiring such knowledge through cross-cultural medical or nursing literature is highly problematic. As Waqar Ahmad (1996, 196) has argued, "The effect of an emphasis entirely on cultural differences to explain inequalities and differences in health status or use of health care services is to pathologize 'culture,' making it the cause of as well as the solution to inequalities in health care."[10] Such uses of "culture" rarely explore the dynamic and contextual aspects of culture or elucidate how attending to culture can obscure other dynamics of racism in the medical setting. The articulation of forms of difference, as Homi Bhabha (1994) argues, is crucial to establishing racial and cultural hierarchies. When called upon to demonstrate such knowledge, the immigrant midwife of colour can never claim the invisible position of "knower," but must always find herself re-inserted into the slot of the "other" who needs to be known. The immigrant midwife of colour, in other words, is instantaneously marginalized when culture is used to articulate difference, even when this is done in the name of "cross-cultural communication."

For one immigrant midwife of colour, navigating the registration process was much easier because she had a close relationship to an established midwifery practice. Before emigrating, she had used her vacation time to visit a midwifery practice in Ontario that her husband's relatives found for her. After immigrating to Canada, she negotiated to become a second attendant in this practice and began the PLEA process. Despite working for minimal remuneration, she felt that her intimate contact with a midwifery practice had given her a significant advantage in the PLEA process:

> Having worked with the midwives here, I felt that there were certain ... luckily, I've had the chance to work with these midwives here because there are certain practices that are different which they expect you to know ... the things that are done here and the things that are done there for different reasons and each person will justify why they do it. Clinical things. I know for sure that here they're very much up on Group B Strep as a major thing, while in [her former country of residence] you just don't check or test for that unless there is a concern ... It's a very major thing here ... So there are certain things that they expect you to know that as a rule, and if you omit it in the exam then you'll be penalized or marks taken away. And there are other little clinical things. I have a list here of all the things that they're checking for and it was very ambiguous ... So luckily for me, I know people who are going through the [Midwifery Education] program so I'd ask them. They're going through the OSCEs [objective structured clinical examinations] and stuff themselves, I'll ask them, "What is it like? What do they expect from you?" (Interview no. 7)

As the immigrant midwives of colour quoted in this section indicate, and as the example of TAAM cited above demonstrates, there was much practical knowledge about midwifery in Ontario that was accessible only to those who had informal access to alternative birth culture or to practising midwives in the province. For numerous reasons, including the outright refusal of admission to those spaces described above, immigrant midwives of colour had little access to knowledge about midwifery that might have facilitated their participation in the PLEA process.

White Behaviours: Encountering the Boundaries of Belonging

Immigrant midwives of colour interviewed for this study identified a number of moments in which they were made to understand that they stood outside the parameters of a normative midwifery identity. Inasmuch as these reminders of difference take place in a context where white women constitute an overwhelming majority, they take on a racial dimension. Practices may be deemed to be racist when they produce subordinations that are "coterminous with 'racially' different populations" (Anthias and Yuval-Davis 1992, 13). In light of this, the effects of being reminded of one's failure to measure up to the norm function differently for racialized minority women than they do for most white women, inasmuch as such a reminder works to reinscribe non-belonging to those for whom non-belonging is already a fact of everyday life. Such inscriptions belong to the arsenal of microexpressions of racialized power. Rarely accomplished through open expressions of racial antipathy, these forms of racial marginalization attach themselves to evaluations of supposedly non-racial characteristics such as speech, deportment, education, and so on, some of which are demonstrated in these narratives.

One native English speaker felt consistently deskilled and inferiorized when her use of language was criticized by Ontario midwives. She was frequently the only woman of colour present at midwifery events she attended, and she talked to me about how she felt when she was in the presence of those midwives who were the first to be registered in the province:

I'm totally incompetent when I put myself against this group. That's how I feel. I'm not. I know I'm not. It's just I come across these midwives ... all the time and some of them I feel, I can't even talk to them. I can't. It's not that I have anything against them, it's not anything like that, it's just the way they are, they way they talk.

I found people correcting the way I spoke, all the time. And so I lost my confidence. I used to tell my husband, it's just the big words that everybody uses. You know, I'm trying to think, just political words. I can't even think. I seem to be able to talk to you okay, but with some people I'll say a sentence and they'll say, "Oh, you mean this" and replace it with a bigger word. You know. I just felt that I had to sort of learn English all over again, you know, learn to sort of express everything in North American language. That's what I have to sort of say to myself, I've never come across that in [her previous country of residence], never.

I was in the midwifery field for at least a good ten years before I came here and all of a sudden I thought ... and so it just made me nervous to speak to people, really. And I suppose it still does, a bit. I just found it very difficult to take part in it because, again, I just thought that the language and everything was so high powered that I was just ... I had nothing to contribute. Whatever I'd say, somebody would alter the way I would say it and I'd feel totally squashed ... By the time the [assessment program for trained midwives] came, I found it quite difficult to even contribute in the sessions because I was so much aware of this "handicap" that I have. (Interview no. 12)

One woman who had succeeded in becoming registered and who knew several people who had failed the PLEA process argued that a lack of white cultural competencies, including the ability to frame interactions within feminist terms and to display political sophistication, was a stumbling block for even the most experienced midwives:

> Some of them [other midwives of colour] couldn't get through because of the way that they talked. I mean how you say it. It's not what you know, it's how you say it. I think that is the main problem. I mean, like so many nurses who work in L & D [labour and delivery] are far better skilled than any of the midwives, I must say, but they fail. And yet they have been doing this ... like [monitoring] fetal distress day in and day out. They fail on *that*. I don't believe it. It's because of the way that they project themselves. "No, this is not the way you speak to *clients*" ... *Middle class, feminism, empower, women's body* and all that is what they want also. It is their downfall. I still visualize being only a midwife and nothing more, but seeing how they work now, you're more than a midwife, you must be very politically oriented as well. (Interview no. 10)

Several of the women interviewed indicated that the impression among immigrant midwives of colour was that midwifery was as an elite white profession geared toward a white clientele and was a milieu in which women of colour would not be welcome. One woman whose work and advocacy activities afforded her contact with many immigrant midwives of colour described her sense of how Ontario midwifery was perceived among that group:

> Actually, most of the people that I talked to they wouldn't even consider applying to do the midwifery even though they're midwifery-trained. Midwives [from the region from which she had emigrated] are double-trained, meaning RN/midwife. And quite a few of them I know were on the labour and delivery. 'Cause I know one lady, she used to work at _____ Hospital, and she says that she would *never* want to do it. She thinks it's, is the word *preppy*? It's a different type of class, she thinks, who goes in to do midwifery and the clientele also; she didn't think it was geared to the clients who would really probably benefit from the midwifery experience. She didn't feel part of the culture. She didn't feel as if this was for *her*. Like it's a different class of people. (Interview no. 13)

Occasionally, reminders of non-belonging were overt. One woman whose experience of a period of supervision in an all-white suburban midwifery practice was highly stressful ("I felt like garbage, like crap," she told me) related that she was told that she should try to advertise herself within her own ethnic community because the clientele in that practice were "too so-phisticated" for her (Interview no. 10). Ironically, in twenty years of prac-tice in her previous country of residence, she had never delivered a woman from her own racialized minority group. Another woman described in great detail an overt reminder of outsider status to which she was subjected dur-ing an encounter with an official from the Prior Learning and Experience Assessment process:

I was *stunned* by the first question ... I sit down and no, no, no ... "What's your name?" and so forth and they say, "Where are you from?" I was stunned! *Where are you from?* She lost me there. I'm sorry, I don't know how I come across to you but I was ... really had an attitude. I said, "Where am I *from!*" I'm sure I said it worse than that. I just did not expect that question. I don't know why. I just did not expect that question. And somehow that was the furthest thing from my mind. It stunned me.

"Where am I from?" What do I say? Do I say, where I'm living here in Canada? Do I say where I'm from in [her country of birth]? Do I say I'm a Canadian citizen? 'Cause I'm sort of used to that type of question. But it is an illegal question, you don't ask people that. I just thought, "This is so inappropriate; what does this have to do with this [event]?" I'm not the only one who feels this way, you know. The girl who came after me in line, she found out and said, "You were angry," and I said, "Oh, my God, did it show?" I *was* angry! I just feel that, oh yeah, I'm failed now because I know I answered the question but I just had a stiff back. Because I spontaneously said, "Where am I *from!* And I actually did this, as to say, "Why are you asking me that?" and "How dare you ask me that!" and "What has this got to do with this [event]?" Anyway, I did answer. I said "I'm a Canadian citi-zen, I'm originally from _____, and I live in _____," whatever. I don't remember if I said that, but I know I said, "I'm a Canadian citizen and I'm originally from _____." Maybe I said three things. But that just threw me off. I just didn't think it was an appropriate question. I don't know, it's like ... a racist question. It *is* a racist question; that's the best way I can describe it. I was uncomfortable and that's when I know that something is not nice. And I felt very uncomfortable. That's the best way to put it. (Inter-view no. 13)

Having entered this particular midwifery-related event prepared to em-phasize her expertise (she is a native English speaker, trained midwife, and seasoned Canadian medical worker), this woman is assaulted with that oft-employed Canadian question "Where are you from?" that conveys to the recipient that she is "other." "To exist," writes Homi Bhabha (1994, 44), "is to be called into being in relation to an otherness, its look or locus" and arguably the question "Where are you from?" performs the "call" in the incident narrated above. The question operates as an engine of differentiation, simultaneously installing the two women in positions of dominance and subordination in relationship to belonging inside the Canadian nation, and inside the midwifery profession. For the white interviewer, the convergence of race and difference is activated when the body of colour enters the room. The question "Where are you from?" guarantees that the woman of colour is "sealed into ... crushing objecthood" (Fanon 1992, 220) in which her status as immigrant person of colour, and the inferiorizing discourses that attach to that status in Canadian society, foreclose prior claims to subjecthood. However, this woman refuses to be sealed into this space on the margins. She realizes the costs, but feels compelled, nonetheless, to exert her subjecthood in the form of a claim to Canadian citizenship as an overriding marker of her identity. An incident such as this may appear accidental but cannot be construed as innocent. Rather, it is an indication not only of how "racializing evaluations" (Goldberg 1993) are used with seeming impunity in everyday situations, but how state institutions such as midwifery help regulate subjects as hierarchically positioned citizens in a world of global migrations (Ong 1996).

Do white immigrant midwives fare better in the PLEA process than their racialized minority colleagues? Anecdotal evidence about who has successfully completed the PLEA process suggests that this is the case. At least one immigrant midwife of colour, a woman who had successfully completed most of the PLEA program, believed that for British-trained midwives of colour the process had been more difficult to navigate than it had been for white British-trained midwives. As Philomena Essed (1991) notes in her study of black women in the Netherlands and the United States, racialized minority women name an experience as "racism" only after every other explanation is rejected as inadequate. Like Essed's subjects, and like other women interviewed for this study, the woman quoted below was hesitant to identify the difficulties of immigrant midwives of colour with racism. However, she ultimately sanctioned this explanation because nothing else can account for the difference she perceives between the experience of women of colour and that of white women immigrants from the UK.[11] This woman, who has had extended contact with PLEA participants, offered this response when asked whether she thought that for some people the PLEA process had been relatively unproblematic:

> I've spoken to a few. I've spoken to a few who said it's okay ... Yes, yes, white British women. And they came over very confident, very masterful people. And they're the kind of people I see within the profession at the moment, very ... almost militant kind of people, you know. Yes, I mean the girls who I ask them what the process is like [and they say], "It's okay, you'll be fine." And "It was piece of cake, it was just a matter of waiting" ...

I have to say, and I don't want to say that there's definite discrimination on their part, but it's very odd that all the – I would say three-quarters of the midwives who expressed dissatisfaction with the process or had problems with the program have been women of colour and then ones that have shown really positive and have found the process not a problem have been white. Definitely for me. And I wasn't looking for that. I wasn't particularly looking for it so it's got to be. (Interview no. 7)

Narratives of Resistance

Despite the fact that antiracism initiatives have been launched to confront inequities in Ontario's health care system, a concerted political effort to counter marginalizing practices was never mounted by, or on behalf of, immigrant midwives of colour wishing to become registered in the province.[12] Indeed, open resistance to these practices might have jeopardized the professional futures of immigrant midwives of colour. However, as Chandra Mohanty (1991) argues, resistance to domination must be understood to occur in forms other than conscious articulation or organized protest, and evidence of resistance needs to be sought in everyday practices. Some of these practices, as Gayatri Spivak (1988) has shown, constitute forms of subaltern speech. However, all speech, claims Spivak (1999, 309), "entails a distanced decipherment by another, which is at best an interception." I am in no way positioned to intercept all evidence of resistant behaviours engaged in by the immigrant midwives of colour interviewed. Because of my dominant positioning in the racial hierarchy, many resistant behaviours and attitudes, no doubt, were never shared with me. And, despite "studying to be political" (Spivak 1999, 378) about the ways that race structures global, local, institutional, and interpersonal dynamics, I will have missed many of the elements of resistance that were articulated in the interviews. However, there are those forms of resistance that I *have* attempted to intercept. Interpretations of resistance and agency must be broadened so that we may see a wider range of actions as constituting resistance to marginalization (Mohanty 1991).

For some women, agreeing to be interviewed constituted a form of resistance, and they offered their narratives as a way to redress, in a public way, some of the wrongs they had themselves experienced. The women of colour who sat on midwifery boards frequently resisted the agenda of white midwives and midwifery activists by arguing for attention to issues of language and access. Immigrant midwives of colour also offered resistant narratives in which they used the discourse of North American childbirth reform to frame their own skills and experience, rendering this expertise commensurate with that of women trained in Ontario. And many, if not most, of the women interviewed continued to refer to themselves as midwives even though the use of that title is proscribed by law for those not registered with the College of Midwives of Ontario.

Resistance inheres in the very willingness to offer a narrative that challenges the "heroic tale" that dominates public discourse around midwifery in Ontario. While many spoke of their admiration for the midwifery project and for those who brought it to fruition, no immigrant midwife of colour interviewed for this study spoke in positive terms when asked the question "Can you tell me about your experience with the PLEA?" The narratives were organized entirely around experiences of exclusion, marginalization, and frustration. One woman who dropped out after completing a significant portion of the PLEA summarized the process as "tough, expensive, time-consuming, stressful and degrading" (Interview no. 3). Several of those interviewed offered broad criticisms of exclusion in the registration process. The women often projected beyond their own experiences of marginalization to encompass those who had access to fewer resources (money, facility in English, etc.) than they did. One native English speaker cited the wasted expertise of those whose ambitions were thwarted because of inadequate performance on the initial language exam. She disputed Ontario midwifery's claims that it is seeking a diverse pool of care providers:

> There were a few people who were in the same situation as me that English was their first language. And there were some people there that English wasn't their first language, but I felt they were fluent enough in English to be able to pass the test. And also I feel that to pass an English proficiency test was a very – if they wanted people from diverse backgrounds, as they say they do, and you know I just feel that the language proficiency test was actually a way of excluding a lot of people. Because even if your first language wasn't English, then if you had the knowledge and the skills and the wherewithal to pass the rest of the assessment that you need to without that, then I feel that the better for the profession, because you need people that have more than one language. Or maybe their English isn't as strong but they're talented and they're good midwives and they can go through the process without maybe having fluent English or can kind of – I don't know what they were expecting really. I just felt that it excluded. Because I was told that half of the people failed and I was surprised about that. (Interview no. 7)

Asked why she thought so few immigrant midwives were practising in Ontario, another PLEA candidate accounted deftly for numerous aspects of exclusion, including lack of financial resources and the need for candidates to possess cultural competencies associated with dominant groups. This woman also criticizes the failure of Ontario midwifery to find Third World "grassroots" midwifery practice – that is community-based, client-centred, low-technology midwifery – commensurable with "grassroots" practice in

Ontario. "Grassroots" status, she implies, is valued only when it describes the origins of white women's activism:

> It's upper-middle-class people who really started this movement. According to my memory, readings. Number two, in the first set of recruitments, they eliminated outsiders. Why they're not there, you're asking? I don't know if I'll finish the process because of finance. I'm working, I have a son. I have my commitment, I have a mortgage. So finance. We're not rich people. I'm thinking about myself here. I'm working, I have to concentrate on my job. It's not like I'm going to go half a day here to study ... Yeah, it's the whole sort of background development. You know, although it's grassroots, for us in [her region of origin] and it's even mentioned, midwifery here is mentioned as grassroots. But what type of grassroots? You know! (Interview no. 13)

Resistance to exclusion can be seen not just in narratives but in women's actions as well. In marked contrast to the Midwifery Education Program, which fosters community-building among students through a week-long, intensive residential workshop at the beginning of the program, as well as through student organizations and everyday contacts, the PLEA process was described by participants as isolating, offering little that would allow women to connect. Nonetheless, some women attempted to build contacts among PLEA participants and personally collected names and addresses of other women of colour they met at AOM or PLEA activities. One woman who made such attempts hinted that although little has come of her efforts so far, the potential for mobilizing women of colour exists:

> When I go to these (PLEA) things I try to take down names, as many as I can so I have names, but we've never done anything with the names as such. Like yesterday I talked to somebody that I met there. But in terms of group activity there hasn't been much. But some people are really stressed by this situation, I feel, and maybe I'm wrong, that they have the energy and it's not being used ... They should be given a medium. (Interview no. 1)

Circulating stories of racism and exclusion constituted another resistance strategy. One women described in detail the rumours of racism within Ontario midwifery that she encountered in 1996 while attempting to maximize her knowledge of childbirth issues through volunteering in labour and delivery departments, attending conferences, and enrolling in academic courses related to women's health:

> I attended many conferences that year, I went to _____ Hospital's two conferences that dealt with women's health and one at the Convention

Centre. So most of the time, whenever I met other women in other positions, especially in the childbirth field, or in [hospital] birthing areas, they talked about this, and from other midwives too, other midwives who have chosen now to practise nursing instead of midwifery. They were saying that ... like the ones I knew were from maybe the Caribbean and Guyana and Jamaica, so most of them were black, so they told me that "because we are black and although we have good experience, they don't want us to go [into midwifery]." And I did a women's health course and I did research actually about midwives and I found that it wasn't just me, that I'm not the only one struggling to get through the PLA. (Interview no. 9)

The discussions of racism that she encountered actually discouraged this woman, who held a recently acquired baccalaureate degree in midwifery from her country of origin, from continuing to pursue registration after she discovered that her PLEA application had been lost by the College of Midwives. Such bureaucratic errors are seldom intentionally racist, but they may be interpreted by racialized minority people as discrimination in light of their experience of racist treatment and of a history of exclusion in Canada. While at the time this woman did not attach racist meanings to her experience with the College of Midwives, circulating stories of racism engendered a reluctance to challenge the bureaucracy that had curtailed her efforts to become registered. As a practising Muslim, she always wore a head scarf in public and she was reluctant, for that reason, to appear in person at the College of Midwives to argue her case. "That was one of the reasons that I didn't push that hard," she explained. "At the time, I was wearing a religious head covering, right? So maybe I didn't have the strength to go ahead because maybe that would be like one of the things, if they are saying that racism is going on, you know, against women of colour ... that was one of the things that has taught me not to go forward" (Interview no. 9).

The circulation of stories describing the midwifery apparatus in Ontario as unwelcoming to women of colour raises once again the issue of how subaltern speech is intercepted and by whom. The small number of women of colour who have succeeded in the PLA/PLEA program and its high attrition rates may be attributed to structural obstacles. However, non-participation must be also read as a form of "speech" that proclaims to whomever is listening that participating in a process that might yield significant rewards may simply not be worth the price of enduring the practices of racist exclusion.

I have traced some of the microprocesses of white dominance that have regulated the participation of women of colour in the establishment of a revitalized midwifery profession in the province of Ontario. I have also attempted, from a vantage point delimited by privilege, to discern some of the resistance strategies employed by those interviewed and others whom they represented in their narratives. What needs to be brought to the foreground is that, in the presence of a significant convergence of philosophy, experience, and education, evidence of the incommensurability between midwives of colour and white midwives was persistently produced not only through policy, but through everyday encounters between women of colour and white women engaged with midwifery in Ontario. The grounds for these claims of incommensurability include the lack of a variety of cultural competencies and inadequate knowledge of local practices and sensibilities, both of which were much more easily available to white midwifery aspirants than to immigrant women of colour. The public articulation of a white racial identity as midwifery's norm was so loud that many women of colour who had had little contact with midwives or the midwifery apparatus in the province perceived themselves as unwanted on midwifery's voyage and chose not to attempt the registration process. The triumph of white women's formulation of midwifery norms and practices was guaranteed by the inferiorization and tokenization of women of colour who attempted to make midwifery practice and service more accessible to racialized minority women in the province.

Seeing the face of racial dominance is a daily occurrence for most people of colour in white-majority contexts. For the racially dominant, however, *not* seeing how such dominance operates unintentionally through the deployment of "epithets, glances, avoidances, characterizations, prejudgements, dispositions, and rationalizations" (Goldberg 1993, 96) is also an everyday occurrence. It has been my intention in this chapter to bring white midwifery's illusion of innocence into conversation with the evidence of harm articulated through words and actions by women of colour who have met the face of white dominance. It is difficult, if not impossible, in the presence of such evidence, to claim that racist effects do not attach themselves to acts that can be rationalized as unrelated to racialized forms of power. "The question," argues Leslie Roman (1993, 73), "is not *whether* the subaltern can speak. Instead, it is whether privileged ... white groups are willing to listen when the subaltern speaks, and how whites can know the difference between occasions for responsive listening and listening as an excuse for silent collusion with the status quo of racial and neocolonial inequalities."

The challenge for those who wish to interrupt such circuits of power is to begin to see those moments when racial meanings are mobilized in and through seemingly neutral acts. Racially dominant people can learn, argues Alison Bailey (1998, 7), "to think and act not out of the 'spontaneous consciousness' of the socially scripted locations that history has written for us, but out of ... traitorous (privilege-cognizant) scripts." Such scripts can never be crafted in isolation but must be authored in partnership with marginalized people and through engagement with theories of antisubordination rooted in collective struggle.

Conclusion:
The Construction of Unequal Subjects

> The important question ... remains whether the emancipatory
> impulse of feminism can only become possible through the
> construction of unequal subjects.
>
> – Inderpal Grewal, "'Women's Rights as Human Rights'"

This book addresses how, given their numbers in the population, immigrant midwives of colour came to be underrepresented in Ontario's newly
legalized midwifery profession. This question has important implications
beyond the immediate context of this book for at least two reasons: (1) If
under-representation such as that described in this book is not natural or
inevitable ("all immigrants require a catching-up time"; "things are fundamentally different here"), then what are the practices that bring it about?
and (2) There is an urgent need to determine, as Inderpal Grewal suggests,
whether feminist emancipatory projects require hierarchical relations. In
other words, does the advancement of white women hinge on the continued subordination of women of colour?

Part of the answer lies in one of the central intentions of this book: to
identify the habits of racial dominance that structure everyday encounters
between white people and racialized minority people so that racially dominant people can begin to recognize, take responsibility for, and ultimately
abandon behaviours that contribute to racial hierarchies. Such a strategy
requires both that stories of subordination be loudly amplified *and* that
those of us on the dominant side of the racial equation attempt to appre-
hend the insurgent responses of subaltern peoples, which have been historically inaudible to us (Spivak 1988). The invocation of racism here is an
unabashedly political move. I mobilize its undeniable discursive power and
moral challenge in the hope that a more intense scrutiny and a swifter
ameliorative process will be brought to bear on the inequities I have worked
to catalogue in these pages.

Being Accountable to the Research Subjects

The question of complicity must also be raised in relationship to my own participation in the systems of domination and subordination outlined in this research. As I mentioned earlier, in one of the interviews I conducted with immigrant women of colour, I became the object of a surprising reversal when the interview subject began to interrogate *me*. In the transcript segment below, I am held accountable for my positioning and for the benefit that the research will yield me, and am forced to explain, in detail, my own motivations, as well as the intentions of my project:

> Interviewee no. 10: The only reason I agreed to do this interview is that ... the paper that you sent me showed that you're not biased ... you know, after reading part of the paper and I thought, "Who is this Sheryl?" If she's white, why does she have to speak up for these ethnic minorities? This intrigues me! That's why I wanted to meet you! What advantage or benefit will *she* get out of this?
>
> Sheryl: That's a very important question that you're asking.
>
> Interviewee no. 10: So, this is the thing, I mean, what is there in it for her? Is she doing it genuinely or is she doing it for something else? I'm being honest. This is my honesty.
>
> Sheryl: They are very important questions and they are questions that I need to answer.
>
> Interviewee no. 10: I thought, well, maybe there's some advantage. Is she going to pursue some other career? I'm being honest.
>
> Sheryl: And I think the honest answer is yes ... There's no question that doing this work gets me a PhD, which may or may not get me a job teaching, which is a very prestigious job and there is a kind of a fad now for antiracism stuff. They want somebody who knows about racism. And it gives me an advantage to be doing this kind of work as opposed to doing something more traditional, standard, right?
>
> Interviewee no. 10: Because you can do any other topic, other than racism.

These questions emphasize the importance of shifting my focus from a concern with textual strategies of accountability to a quest for more perceptibly material ones. This woman asks if my engagement with this research is a "genuine" one, and I interpret genuineness here to mean a commitment to circulating the data effectively as a tool for change rather than using them only as an instrument for professional and personal advancement. How, it must be asked, do I envision my responsibility for the knowledge I have produced in these pages? If this book is not to serve simply as a vehicle for conferring status and authority on its author, and for positioning white people once again as "the heroic agents of racism's decline" (Weigman 1995, 2), what course should I pursue? I can only suggest some of the ways I can carry out the promise of accountability with which I undertook and negotiated interviews with all of those who, by agreeing to be interviewed, took considerable risks.

First, I must emphasize that after the anti-oppression theories have been foregrounded, the unanticipated connections traced, and the broad conclusions drawn, nothing about the relationships of inequality can be said to have changed in any substantial way. We are left instead with an identifiable set of unequal relationships, attendant material inequities, and a trail of individual and collective indignities, which cannot be resolved through even the most thorough cataloguing. Interventions such as this one can only hope to have effects if they receive enough public exposure to actually interrupt circulating discourses. The data contained here, for example, may be of use to community activists and those in non-governmental agencies who struggle with equity issues related to internationally educated professionals. It is clear that prior learning assessment programs, while ostensibly more flexible and equitable than other forms of credentials assessment, are not exempt from racist processes. This work might provide ways of talking about the racist effects of bureaucratic procedures and intersubjective encounters on immigrant people of colour. I also believe that insurgent voices in the midwifery community require the documentation of racist and other exclusionary processes that this study offers, in order to make concrete a public struggle for equity.

There is a final reason that makes distribution of these findings critically important if I am to be accountable to the women who have participated in this research. My intent is to bring Ontario midwifery's illusion of innocence into direct contact with evidence of the harm that racial dominance enacts. Indeed, what is due to those who shared their stories with me is the creation of an historical record that makes continued ignorance of racist exclusions and other inequalities a form of wilful ignorance and that consequently renders ongoing discriminatory practices deliberate and indefensible.

There is some evidence that the white midwives and their supporters who have until recently been heedless of the racist exclusion that underpins the re-emergence of midwifery have begun to acknowledge this lamentable history.[1] There are also profound changes happening in the recognition of international credentials in Canada. Since I began this research in 1995, there has been a groundswell of public concern over how immigrants' skills are undervalued and a growing realization that refusal to recognize foreign credentials is a human rights issue (Cornish, McIntyre, and Pask 2001). Despite the groundbreaking work accomplished by the 1989 *Access!* report submitted by the Task Force on Access to Professions and Trades in Ontario, most of its recommendations were never adopted as government policy (Policy Roundtable Mobilizing Professions and Trades [PROMPT] 2004, 14). However, community-based advocacy groups, immigrant services groups, and non-governmental funding agencies, as well as an access-focused group formed by the province's twelve occupational regulatory bodies, including the College of Midwives, have in recent years invested considerable time and effort into developing solutions to these problems.[2] While some of these solutions hold promise, there is still a need to assess both the proposed strategies and those currently being implemented for their discriminatory impact (PROMPT 2004, 29).[3] In implementing its Immigration and Refugee Protection Act in 2002, Canada has shifted from privileging occupational criteria for admission to an emphasis on skills, experience, age, and competence (Kofman 2004, 655). Aimed at alleviating labour shortages in developed countries, this process may open the nation's portals to foreign-trained professionals, but it proceeds to absorb them, unevenly, into a racially segmented labour force.

Race blindness enabled almost every exclusionary policy and process documented in these pages. When race is not addressed directly and consistently as a factor that operates to give women different and unequal lives, then racism inevitably is reproduced. Because the Ontario midwifery movement understood its project as one that would benefit all women equally, it could and did avoid recognizing that women's stakes in the politics of midwifery reflected the ways in which they were positioned by race. Messages emphasizing that race mattered, even when spoken directly by racialized minority women, remained inaudible to those who pursued the re-emergence of the profession. As a consequence, the movement to legalize midwifery could not and did not avoid enacting racist exclusion.

Documenting the macroprocesses and microprocesses that produce and reproduce inequality has been key here. White women's mobility in the West has been enabled by the available labour of Third World migrant women who are often channelled into jobs that white women have abandoned. This process frequently involves the significant deskilling of migrant professionals. The presence in the health care sector in Ontario of substantial numbers of immigrant women of colour and the exodus from nursing of non-immigrant women is a case in point.

The midwifery apparatus participated in this deskilling of immigrants of colour and in the construction of a local racial hierarchy by putting into place policies that rendered the professional training and other competencies of immigrant women of colour inadequate. Even those midwives of colour who had extensive and parallel professional preparation in their countries of origin, who spoke English as a first language or adequately as a second language, and who had had unblemished midwifery careers – sometimes of more than twenty years' duration – found that the exceedingly high cost of assessment procedures, the demands for additional baccalaureate credentials, and requirements in terms of time away from work and family made the continued pursuit of a midwifery career in Canada untenable. Only two of the ten women interviewed who had participated in the PLA/PLEA process have become eligible for registration.

Resources such as financial aid, and personal and academic support systems such as those developed for white students who were being groomed as the "ambassadors to the profession," were glaringly absent from the process through which immigrant women of colour passed. Those who chose to participate in this process encountered numerous additional obstacles including a lack of access to practising midwives and to relationships where knowledge of local conventions of practice might be acquired, reinforcement of their outsider status through references to national origin and to "inadequate" cultural competencies, and unintentional bureaucratic errors and delays. Never intentionally racist nor clearly discriminatory by liberal standards, these practices and policies nonetheless created racist effects because their impact was more negative for women of colour than it was for white women.

Future Research

Data about white immigrant midwives, including those from Eastern, Southern, and Western Europe, were not included in this study. However, anecdotal evidence indicates that this group has been more successful in entering the midwifery profession in Ontario through the College of Midwives' Prior Learning and Experience Assessment program than have immigrant women of colour. It is possible to speculate that the experience of "near white" groups such as Eastern European immigrants might yield particularly interesting data on how race operates to produce exclusions and inclusions. A more detailed comparison of how white immigrant women and immigrant women of colour have fared in the PLA/PLEA program could shed light on the processes by which white immigrants make social and material gains that situate them far more advantageously in the Canadian social matrix than visible minority immigrants (Lian and Matthews 1998).

Insurgent Possibilities: How Things Change

> Full of voice, she slipped out of the velvety darkness that was her
> mother's womb, into the light. I was overcome. I watched as
> Qwyn, this tiny golden-umber coloured soul, caught by an
> opaque rubber gloved doctor, in a white coat, was separated from
> the placenta and bundled into blanched cloth. I stood there for a
> moment and wondered how she would come to know of herself,

blinded by the glare of snow? What would this fair world tell her?
I experienced such a sadness for her – or maybe it was for myself.

– Djanet Sears, "Notes of a 'Coloured Girl'"

Birth is a critically important event and I would have liked to have explored some of the insurgent, recuperative, and antiracist possibilities of a racially diverse midwifery community. For those doing research at the nexus of race, gender, and nation, as well as for those who care about the pernicious effects of racism, there are pressing questions to ask about whose reproduction is supported and celebrated and whose reproduction is contained and regulated.[4] Racism is alive and well in Canada – it should not come as a surprise that the act of producing racialized minority babies within a white-majority society might engender no less an uneasy white response than does the entrance into Canada of immigrants of colour. There already exists convincing evidence that women of colour endure specific forms of gendered racism when they deliver their babies in Canadian hospitals.[5]

I have no clear ideas about how racialized minority midwives might be able to use midwifery care to mitigate the messages of white moral authority and cultural dominance that may be transmitted during childbirth. I do, however, continue to have faith in the model of a community-controlled out-of-hospital birth centre – acknowledging the many erasures that the concept of "community" enacts – that pursues hiring policies and adopts practices that privilege rather than penalize immigrant midwives of colour and provides a space for consciously reconfiguring the childbearing experiences of marginalized women. I believe that having few immigrant midwives of colour makes the possibility of recuperating birth from racist practices less likely. This lack of immigrant midwives of colour, I would argue, renders the midwifery establishment complicit in a system of racial dominance that, as Djanet Sears (1997) describes so poetically, leaves its imprint from the moment of birth.

Accounting for Our "Bloody Genealogies"
In response to the question posed by Inderpal Grewal (1999) – "whether the emancipatory impulse of feminism can only become possible through the construction of unequal subjects" – I must answer that the evidence gathered here substantiates her suspicion that feminist imperatives are impossibly modernist constructs firmly grounded in the construction of unequal subjects. Unequal relations between immigrant midwives of colour and white midwives, and between Third World women and Ontario midwives, remain firmly in place even as the re-emergence of midwifery is hailed as a "victory for women." Such an outcome, it seems, is unavoidable when, in the course of formulating our feminist projects, those of us

in dominant positions insist on our innocent positioning and fail to account for what Jane Flax (1998, 142) has deemed the "bloody genealogies" of our subjectivities. If there is even a glimmer of hope for constructing political projects that do not reproduce hierarchical relations among women and other pernicious effects of modernity, then such genealogies and the material and discursive conditions from which they spring must be the subject of a painful but necessary accounting.

Appendices

Appendix A: Information Letter for Research Participants

Dear [name of potential participant],
I am a student at the Ontario Institute for Studies in Education of the University of Toronto currently working on my PhD dissertation, entitled "Obstructed Labour: Race and Gender in the Re-emergence of Midwifery in Ontario." In my work, I am researching how different groups have participated in, and benefited differently from, the movement to legalize midwifery. This letter is intended to invite your participation in an interview that will provide material for part of my dissertation.

Participation in this research will allow you to contribute to an interpretation of the history of the midwifery movement. If you have played a policy-making role, it will offer you a chance to interpret why and how various decisions affected different social groups. If you have an interest in practising midwifery and have not been given an opportunity to do so in the province, participation in this research offers you a chance to discuss your relationship as a trained midwife to the process by which midwifery has become legal and to discuss the current state of midwifery in the province as it affects you.

While I am a long-time supporter of the midwifery model of care, and this study is not intended in any way to raise doubts about or to undermine the importance of that model, it will raise questions about how successful the midwifery movement in Ontario has been in making midwifery practice accessible to a diverse group of women. It is important for you to know that your participation will contribute to an analysis that may be critical of the political decisions of the midwifery movement.

If you agree to be interviewed, you will be asked to sign a "Letter of Consent to Participate in Research," in which you agree to have any remarks you make in the interview recorded and used in my dissertation and in any articles or books I may write about my work.

Prior to my preparation of the dissertation, you will be sent a transcript of the interview and if you believe that your views have not been accurately represented on the tape, you may contact me so that clarification can be made. Your anonymity is of utmost concern to me and I will take special precautions not to include information that would allow you to be identified in my work unless you choose to be identified. Using categories that I provide, you will be asked to indicate on the transcript how you would like me to identify the source of all quotations that come from our interview. On completion of the work, I will be happy to make a copy available to you if you so wish. It is important to understand that while I undertake to express your ideas accurately, the written report of this research may contain criticism of your opinions or remarks.

At every point, your anonymity will be maintained. Copies of the questionnaires, tapes, and transcripts in my possession will be kept locked up and may be accessed only by me, my thesis advisor, Prof. Sherene Razack, and members of my thesis committee, Prof. Ruth

Roach Pierson and Prof. Kari Dehli. These documents will be labelled with code names that will also be used to refer to you in any written report. At your request, your contribution can be deleted from the tapes and transcripts following the submission of my thesis. *You may withdraw from the study at any point.*

Please accept my thanks for your willingness to participate in this project.

Appendix B: Poster Posted in the Labour and Delivery Departments of Two Toronto Hospitals, to Solicit Study Participants

Are you a *trained midwife* from the Caribbean, China, the Philippines, Africa, the Middle East or South Asia?

I am a doctoral student at the University of Toronto doing research for my dissertation, which analyzes barriers to access to the midwifery profession in Ontario. I am interested in interviewing women trained in midwifery from the Caribbean, China, the Philippines, Africa, the Middle East or South Asia. I am particularly interested in interviewing labour and delivery/postpartum nurses who have interacted with Ontario-trained midwives over the past ten years.

Interviews typically last 1-1½ hours, are tape recorded and can be conducted anywhere and at any time which is convenient to you. Extreme care is being taken to protect the identities of those interviewed. This research is supported by a Doctoral Fellowship awarded by the Social Science and Humanities Research Council of Canada.

Appendix C: Chronology of the Re-Emergence of Midwifery in Ontario

1973   Ontario Nurse-Midwives Association (ONMA) founded
1976   Home Birth Task Force formed
1981   Ontario Association of Midwives (OAM) formed
1982   Coroner's inquest into baby death in Kitchener-Waterloo area
       College of Physicians and Surgeons of Ontario bans physician participation in home birth
       Health Professions Legislation Review (HPLR) begins
1983   Midwifery Task Force of Ontario (MTFO), a midwifery consumer group, formed
       Joint submission of the OAM and ONMA to the HPLR
1985   Association of Ontario Midwives (AOM) formed through merger of OAM and ONMA
       Coroner's inquest into baby death on Toronto Island
       HPLR recommends incorporation of midwifery into Ontario's health care system
1986   Task Force on the Implementation of Midwifery in Ontario (TFIMO) appointed by Ministry of Health
1987   Publication of Report of the Task Force on the Implementation of Midwifery in Ontario
1989   Interim Regulatory Council on Midwifery (IRCM) appointed by Minister of Health
       Curriculum Design Committee (CDC) appointed by Minister of Health
1990   First reading in the Ontario Legislature of the Midwifery Act
       Midwifery Integration Planning Project (MIPP) launched
1992   Michener Institute Pre-registration Program for practising midwives begins
1993   February – Transitional Council of the College of Midwives of Ontario appointed
       September – Midwifery Education Program begins in three Ontario universities; Community Advisory Committee to the Prior Learning Assessment project established
       October – sixty-three midwives graduate from Michener Institute program; Committee for More Midwives organizes; Association for Philippine Midwives forms
       December 31 – proclamation of Midwifery Act, 1991; Transitional Council becomes College of Midwives of Ontario (CMO)
1994   First cycle of Prior Learning Assessment (PLA) launched

1996 First class of the Midwifery Education Program graduates
1997 Second Cycle of Prior Learning and Experience Assessment (PLEA) launched

Appendix D: Interview Schedule for Immigrant Midwives of Colour

1 Can you tell me something about your background. Where and when did you grow up? Can you tell me something about your socioeconomic and educational background?
2 When and why did you decide to become a midwife?
3 Can you tell me about the training process that you underwent to become a midwife. What is your personal philosophy of midwifery?
4 Please tell me about the work of midwives in your country of origin. How do they fit into the medical care system? Did you do prenatal and postpartum care? Did you attend home births?
5 When you came to Canada, did you know what the state of midwifery practice was at the time?
6 When did you first hear about the Ontario midwifery movement? What did you think about it at the time?
7 Did you ever participate in activities or organizations which worked for the legalization of midwifery in Ontario? If yes, which ones, when, and in what capacity? What was your experience of these organizations? If no, why didn't you participate?
8 Ivy Bourgeault (1996) has described an "elite" of midwives who were at the centre of midwifery activism. How would you position yourself in relation to this group?
9 In the course of your involvement with midwifery in Ontario, do you recall the participation of other women of colour? What can you tell me about their participation?
10 Why did you decide to pursue/not to pursue registration? IF SUBJECT DID NOT PURSUE REGISTRATION, GO TO QUESTION 13; IF SUBJECT SOUGHT REGISTRATION OR HAD PREREGISTRATION EXPERIENCE:
11 Can you tell me how you came to participate in the Michener/PLA/PLEA. What was your experience of this process?
12 What percentage of your own clientele, in the years prior to legislation, consisted of women of colour? Now?
13 Given that nearly half of all the women who have expressed an interest in practising midwifery since 1987 are visible minority women, how do you understand the current situation in which just 5 percent of midwives in the province are Aboriginal women or women of colour?

Appendix E: Interview Schedule for White "Non-elite" Midwives

1 Can you tell me something about your background. Where and when did you grow up? Can you tell me something about your socioeconomic and educational background?
2 When and how did you become involved in midwifery?
3 What was your experience of the Michener Institute Pre-registration Program?
4 Is there anything about your personal style, your history, etc., that might be seen to be in conflict with the image that the midwifery movement has wanted to project since the struggle for legalization began?
5 Have you participated in any groups that have worked for the legalization of midwifery? Which ones? In what capacity?
6 How would you describe the people with whom you have worked in the midwifery movement? What demographic/social/educational characteristics did you seem to share? How did differences manifest themselves within the movement?
7 Ivy Bourgeault (1996) has described an "elite" of midwives who were at the centre of midwifery activism. How would you position yourself in relation to this group?
8 In the course of your midwifery activism, do you recall the participation of any women of colour? What can you tell me about their participation?

9 What percentage of your own clientele, in the years prior to legislation, consisted of women of colour? Now?
10 Did you ever leave the country to gain midwifery expertise? Where did you go? Can you describe the setting, clientele, working conditions, etc.? How do you feel your experience influenced your status as a midwife in Ontario? Did you go abroad to obtain birth numbers for admission to the Michener Institute program?
11 Given that nearly half of all the women who have expressed an interest in practising midwifery since 1987 are visible minority women, how do you understand the current situation in which just 5 percent of midwives in the province are Aboriginal women or women of colour?

Appendix F: Interview Schedule for White Members of Midwifery Bodies

1 Can you tell me something about your background and about what you do now?
2 Can you tell me about your relationship to midwifery in Ontario?
3 What bodies have you served on and when were you appointed to them? How did you come to be appointed? How long did you serve?
4 What specific issues were you involved with in the legalization process?
5 How did [the body served on] understand the issue of "foreign-trained" midwives? Which committees/members addressed this issue? What positions did they take?
6 How, in your estimation, did the recommendation of the Task Force on the Implementation of Midwifery that candidates for the Midwifery Integration Project (Michener Institute) be resident in the province for twelve months prior to the program get finalized as a requirement that midwives had to have *practised* in the province in the period prior to regulation?
7 What is your understanding of the professional and demographic composition of the IRCM/TC/CMO?
8 Did specific issues relating to "equity" arise in the IRCM/TC/CMO? What were they? Who raised them? How were they addressed?
9 Given that nearly half of all the women who have expressed an interest in practising midwifery since 1987 are visible minority women, how do you understand the current situation in which just 5 percent of midwives in the province are aboriginal women or women of colour?

Appendix G: Interview Schedule for Women of Colour Who Participated on Midwifery Bodies

1 Please tell me something about your background and about what you do now.
2 When and how did you get involved with the midwifery movement in Ontario?
3 Please tell me about your participation. Did you go to meetings, etc.? How often, where, and with whom?
4 What were your expectations for the participation of immigrant midwives of colour in midwifery here? '
5 Have you spoken with them about this process?
6 How do you explain their absence?
7 How do you think they should proceed? What might change things?

Notes

Introduction: A New Profession to the White Population in Canada

1 Putt was later known as Betty-Anne Daviss.

2 The four routes available for those wishing to enter the midwifery profession have included (1) a one-time "grandparenting-in" process made available to some practising midwives in the period immediately prior to the legal proclamation of midwifery in Ontario on 31 December 1993; (2) a four-year baccalaureate program currently offered at three Ontario universities; and (3) the College of Midwives of Ontario's Prior Learning Assessment and subsequent Prior Learning and Experience Assessment program, which processed three cohorts of foreign-trained midwives between 1995 and 2001; and (4) a newly revamped International Midwives Pre-registration Program offered at Ryerson University's School of Continuing Education in partnership with the College of Midwives of Ontario and the Midwifery Education Programme – Ontario Consortium (Laurentian, McMaster, and Ryerson universities). Funding for this bridging program is provided by the Ontario Ministry of Training, Colleges and Universities.

3 These figures do not necessarily reflect the actual number of women of colour who have succeeded in becoming employed as midwives in the province.

4 The terminology surrounding the classification of midwives is complex, and it shifts depending on geographical and temporal location. The use of the term "lay midwifery" here is meant to invoke the context during which that term was current, and to identify midwives who may have been trained in formal training programs and through empirical means but who are not affiliated with nurse-midwifery or direct-entry midwifery training in medical institutions. Its use, however, has for some time been considered to be disrespectful of the considerable expertise of those midwifery practitioners educated outside of medical institutions and it has come to be replaced by the designation "direct-entry midwife," a term I employ in this book. Direct-entry midwifery in Canada and the United States largely refers to midwives who are institutionally educated but who have not been required to undergo prior nursing training. For a discussion of the different usages of classifying terms for midwives see Rooks (1997, 8).

5 While some of the goals of traditional and feminist women's health movements converge, including concern with humane and respectful medical care, appropriate use of medical technology, and informed choice in health care decision-making, their ideological positions on a variety of issues, including access to abortion and women's relationship to the family, differ widely. For critical perspectives on traditional women's health movements see, for example, Gorham and Andrews (1990). On feminist women's health movements in Canada, see Kleiber and Light (1978); Dua et al. (1994); and Adams and Bourgeault (2003). On the 1960s counterculture's effects on the childbirth reform movement, see Umansky (1996). For an excellent chronology of childbirth reform in the United States, see Shearer (1989). For an examination of childbirth reform in Canada in the 1970s and 1980s, see Romalis (1985).

6 Medical misogyny must be understood to have significant racial dimensions. What I am attempting to characterize here is how childbirth reform has been couched primarily in gender terms. For a rare exception, see Waite (1993).

7 The term "women of colour" in its various forms is a problematic but indispensable one. While this phrase represents an act of self-definition and resistance to racist terminology by groups that have been subjected to racialized definitions and exclusions, it nonetheless fails to capture the multiple subject positions occupied by these women. In some senses the term represents the inadequacy of contemporary language in representing multiply constituted identities, a condition Ali Rattansi (1994, 59) has called "a perennial excess of things over words."

8 Unlike physicians in the rest of the country, Ontario's doctors did not oppose legalized midwifery, but they did stridently oppose home birth, a practice that midwives considered key to autonomous midwifery practice and one they refused to abandon under the proposed legislation.

9 Midwifery is currently regulated by legislation in the following provinces: British Columbia, Alberta, Saskatchewan, Manitoba, Ontario, and Quebec. Legislation was introduced in 2003 to regulate midwifery in the Northwest Territories.

10 The use of the term "Third World" continues to demand explication. The assertion of Theo David Goldberg (1993, 155) that "Third World" is one of three "conceptual schemata hegemonic in the production of contemporary racialized knowledge that now define and order popular conceptions of people racially conceived," and that of Ella Shohat and Robert Stam that First World/Third World struggles take place not only *between* nations but also *within* them must be acknowledged. With this in mind, I adopt this term as a provisional one. As Shohat and Stam (1994, 26) argue, "Third World" can signal "both the dumb inertia of neocolonialism and the energizing collectivity of radical critique but with the caveat that the term obscures fundamental issues of race, class, gender and culture."

11 While in the prelegislation period, white midwives and midwifery aspirants travelled with some frequency to Third World sites seeking midwifery experience, in recent years, First Nations midwives from Ontario have also pursued midwifery training in clinics on the Texas-Mexico border, choosing to circumvent the provincial midwifery education and certification programs. Such a development raises complex and difficult questions about the hierarchical relationships among marginalized First World and Third World women.

12 *Shiksa* is a Yiddish term for a gentile or non-Jewish woman.

13 There is not adequate space here to demonstrate the degree to which the benefits accruing to Jews through assimilation have been accompanied by exorbitant costs, including the constant reformulation of gender and ethnic identities to bring them more into line with white Protestant norms (Prell 1999).

14 In her dissertation, Margaret Macdonald (1999, 14) reports that my research has been characterized by midwives in Ontario as "harsh," "inaccurate," and "premature."

15 The reaction of some faculty members in the Midwifery Education Program should not be viewed as representative of the response my research has elicited within the white midwifery community. Some veteran white midwives have been supportive of my work and continue to give me encouragement and feedback. However, the most enthusiastic support has come from midwifery students who have contacted me to discuss my work. Midwifery students have demonstrated a significant degree of resistance to white dominance in midwifery and have organized antiracism initiatives in both the Ryerson University and McMaster University midwifery education program sites (Nestel 1996/7).

16 In the fall of 1996, the Toronto Birth Centre committee was preparing to implement a project, twenty years in the making, for a community-controlled, out-of-hospital childbearing centre based on principles of access, equity, and the appropriate use of technology (Sutton, Cheetham, Krieger, and Sternberg 1993). The result of tens of thousands of hours of volunteer labour, the project was cut by the newly elected Progressive Conservative government in Ontario. As a board member, it fell to me and several others to dismantle the organization's massive archives. What came into my hands was a wealth of historical data documenting the re-emergence of midwifery in Ontario, including newsletters, re-

ports, personal correspondence, announcements of events, and minutes of meetings. Having direct access to these documents was important inasmuch as I felt that organizations such as the AOM and the College of Midwives might deny me full access to their archives because of the controversial nature of my research.

Forty-nine women were originally interviewed; two women withdrew from the study. The interviews were conducted between December 1997 and February 1999 and lasted between forty-five minutes and four hours each. I transcribed all the interviews. The nine hundred pages of interview data were then coded using QSR NUD*IST (Qualitative Solutions and Research, Non-numerical Unstructured Data Indexing, Searching and Theorizing) computer software. For a discussion of NUD*IST software in qualitative analysis see Pateman (1998).

17 Themes were determined separately for the following groups of interview subjects: white midwifery board members, board members of colour, white non-elite practising midwives, white non-practising midwives, white midwifery students, midwifery students of colour, immigrant midwives of colour who participated in the College of Midwives' postlegislation Prior Learning and Experience Assessment program or its prelegislation Michener Institute Midwifery Integration Planning Program, immigrant midwives of colour who did not participate in the Prior Learning and Experience Assessment process, and African-American midwives in the United States.

18 All of the interviews I conducted with immigrant midwives of colour who were not previously known to me took place in their homes in the Greater Toronto Area, largely in the eastern and western suburbs of the city. The one remaining interview took place in a shopping mall in Eastern Ontario.

19 I also attempted to solicit interviews beyond my personal contacts. A leaflet was posted for me in several hospital labour and delivery departments in the Toronto area by nurses with whom I was acquainted. See Appendix B.

20 In identifying the interviews, I use numbers (Interview no. 1, Interview no. 2, etc.) to avoid assigning or having participants choose names that might, through being linked to an ethnic identity, inadvertently make the participant more likely to be recognized.

21 Students reported being overwhelmed with requests from social science researchers for interviews and indicated that they had become reluctant to grant them.

22 I have standardized the English usage in material taken from the interviews with women for whom English was not a first language. Nuance and creative uses of language will have been lost. However, given that English testing has been the most formidable barrier facing immigrant midwives of colour, I thought that displaying any non-standard English usage might function to inferiorize them undeservedly. (In only one case did I feel that communication was less than satisfactory owing to a language barrier.) In the quoted interviews an ellipsis indicates a pause in the narrative and an ellipsis contained in brackets [...] indicates a place where text was excised for clarity or brevity.

23 Two employees of the College of Midwives did meet with me in 1998 to clarify aspects of the Prior Learning and Experience Assessment program.

24 While I will use the term "Ontario midwives" to designate the predominantly white group that practised midwifery outside of the medical system and organized the profession's legalization campaign, I acknowledge the contradictory nature of the term. I would argue that midwives trained outside the province who wish to practise but who are not registered also need to be regarded as "Ontario midwives" (although they are legally proscribed from using that term), inasmuch as they have undergone formal training and are residents of the province.

Chapter 1: Technologies of Exclusion

1 The Live-in Caregiver Program (formerly the Foreign Domestic Movement Program) was initiated in 1981 to recruit female migrant workers to Canada as live-in domestics and nannies (Bakan and Stasiulis 1994, 10).

2 For examples of Canadian scholarship on this subject, see Pratt (1999); Bakan and Stasiulis (1994, 1997, 2004); Daenzer (1993); Macklin (1992); Arat-Koc (1989); and Silvera (1989). For a historical perspective, see Calliste (1991).

3 In 1982, the Canadian Nurses Association adopted what has become known as the "Entry to Practice" position (Baumgart and Larsen 1992, 392). While the position stipulated that the preferred basic credential of nurses entering practice in the year 2000 and beyond be a baccalaureate degree in nursing, this policy has yet to be implemented in all Canadian provinces (Canadian Nurses Association 2003). At present, approximately 23 percent of currently practising registered nurses (RNs) have a baccalaureate nursing degree (Natural Resources Canada 2004). More than half of recent nursing graduates are baccalaureate prepared (Canadian Institute for Health Information 2004), whereas in 1989, just 14 percent of RNs were baccalaureate-prepared (Sedivy-Glasgow 1992, 28). A university degree continues to represent an elite attainment for women in Canada, where only 12 percent of all women have completed a bachelor's degree or higher degree (Statistics Canada 2003).

4 The term "foreign-trained" is a contested one, inasmuch as the word "foreign" is used to describe what is considered alien or unnatural. As such, it reinforces xenophobic notions of immigrants' inferior status. The many groups that have begun to advocate for the recognition of credentials gained outside Canada have adopted the term "internationally educated," which although imprecise at least challenges the pejorative effect of "foreign-trained." For the most part, I will use the term "foreign-trained" here, as it reflects the terminology in use during the period under examination and more precisely captures the exclusionary policies and attitudes I am attempting to document.

5 Economists have argued that immigrants from Third World countries represent a significant source of highly skilled labour for Canada (Akbar and Devoretz 1993; Badets and Howatson-Leo 1999; Antunes, MacBride-King, and Swettenham 2004). Immigrant midwives of colour (most of whom also have nursing training) are part of the phenomenon of a medical brain drain from the South, which is embedded in specific neocolonial economic conditions. Estimates of the number of nurses who have left the Philippines to work in other countries indicate that almost 70 percent of the total nursing labour force of 130,000 has sought work elsewhere (Chang 1997, 137; Gonzales 1992, 23; Ortin 1990, 340). Nearly 20 percent of all hospital-employed registered nurses in New York City come from Asia, with the vast majority coming from the Philippines (Ong and Azores 1994, 182). An astonishing 95 percent of Jamaica's professional nurses migrated between 1975 and 1985, predominantly to the United States and Canada (Deere et al. 1990, 77).

As Cynthia Enloe (1989, 184) has pointed out, "International debt politics has helped create the incentives for many women to emigrate, while at the same time it has made governments dependent on the money those women send home to their families." Remittances sent by migrant workers and immigrants account for a sizeable proportion of the gross domestic product of supplier countries. The Philippines, for example, receives over US$2.9 billion yearly in remittances from migrant labourers, making migrant labour its primary source of foreign currency and a critical resource for servicing its international debt (Chang 1997, 136). The export of skilled professionals such as nurses is yet another way that poorer countries subsidize the high standard of living in economically advantaged ones: high training costs associated with producing skilled labour are paid by sender countries while receiver countries benefit (Sassen 1988, 39).

6 In 1989 more than half the positions for pharmacists, medical technologists, registered nurses, nursing assistants, and public health inspectors went unfilled in the Jamaican health care system (French 1994, 169). A similar situation exists in the Philippines, where almost two-thirds of trained nurses have migrated to work abroad since 1990 (Ball 2004, 125). The lack of nurses has created a burden on those remaining as they endure heavier workloads, overtime, absenteeism, burnout, and increased illness (Ortin 1990; Ong and Azores 1994; Ball 2004). Migration politics have driven curriculum design in Philippines nursing schools since the early twentieth century when American colonial educational policies restructured nursing training in the Philippines to conform to the American model (Choy 2003). Graduates, who began migrating to the United States in the tens of thousands by the 1950s, were trained in the predominantly hospital-based curative nursing model suitable to health care systems in industrialized nations rather than in rural and community preventive practice appropriate to the needs of many Filipinos (Ortin 1990, 341; Ball 2004, 132).

7 Such a pattern is discernible in Canadian women's employment trends in recent years. There is evidence that more Canadian women have been able to move into what were formerly male-dominated (as well as more lucrative and prestigious) professions. There has been a sizeable increase, for example, in the percentage of female physicians and dentists in Canada, which rose from 44 percent in 1987 to 54 percent in 2002 (Cooke-Reynolds and Zukewich 2004). Between 1971 and 1987 the number of women in engineering rose from 1.2 percent of all graduates to 12.2 percent, and in the legal profession, the increase was from 9.4 percent to 47.7 percent (Statistics Canada 1990, 50).

8 Unpublished Statistics Canada data from the 1991 Census provide a broad picture of the how those nurses described as members of "visible minorities" participated in the nursing labour force at the beginning of the 1990s. Out of a total of 89,725 RNs in Ontario, 14.3 percent (12,845) were members of "visible minority" groups. Of the 19,560 licensed practical nurses (LPNs, formerly known as registered nursing assistants) 12.4 percent (2,430) were members of racial minorities. While RNs and LPNs of colour constituted 17.5 percent of the total nursing labour force in the province, only 7.8 percent (490) of head nurses belonged to a racial minority. Seventy-five percent of RNs and LPNs worked in the Toronto Census Metropolitan Area. The provincial statistics are, therefore, of little use in understanding the participation of nurses of colour in nursing labour in Toronto, where 32.8 percent (9,685) of registered nurses and 37.8 percent (1,835) of registered nursing assistants were nurses of colour. In Toronto, where nurses of colour made up 33.5 percent of the total nursing population, they accounted for only 18 percent (340) of head nurses (Statistics Canada 1991a; 1991b).

   Recent data indicate that RN immigration increased from 1999-2002 and that the more than 45,000 registered nurses who immigrated in those years represented 21.8 percent of all immigrants listed under health professions (Bauman et al. 2004, 18). Nearly 40 percent of RNs immigrated from the Philippines, Hong Kong, India, or Jamaica, indicating that a substantial percentage of these nurses are people of colour. Nearly 30 percent of RNs immigrating to Canada come from the United Kingdom, which has historically been the sending country for a substantial proportion of nurses of colour (Stasiulis and Bakan 2003, 116), likely increasing the total percentage of recent immigrant RNs of colour. Further statistical research needs to be done in order to clarify how different racial/ethnic groups are currently situated within the nursing labour force.

9 The Midwifery Act had its first reading in the Ontario Legislature in June of 1990, therefore the period covered in this section spans the very first stirrings of midwifery re-emergence in the mid-1970s to the first reading of the Midwifery Act.

10 For an analysis of the move from home to hospital birth in the United States, see Wertz and Wertz (1989). For a discussion of this phenomenon in Canada, see Arnup (1994).

11 For a detailed account of the political movement to legalize midwifery in Ontario, see Bourgeault (1996). For a description of midwives and midwifery in Ontario between 1960 and 1987, see Fynes (1994).

12 "Activism" in the case of those interviewed varies. Some white midwives interviewed were active members of the Ontario Association of Midwives and later the Association of Ontario Midwives; others confined their participation to attending workshops and conferences or participating in wider childbirth-reform activities. While most of those interviewed would not define themselves as among the most politically active of midwives, all interviewees participated in midwifery-related activities in the province and would have had occasion to meet and interact with women involved in the re-emergence of midwifery from across the province.

13 In November of 1982 the provincial Conservative government announced the formation of a Health Professions Legislation Review, which was to construct a new regulatory framework for governing the health professions. The HPLR was to recommend to the government which health professions needed to be regulated, how the existing Health Disciplines Act was to be revised, what new structures were needed to govern health professions, and which outstanding issues needed resolution (Bourgeault 1996, 79).

14 This organization is entirely separate and distinct from the provincial Task Force on the Implementation of Midwifery in Ontario, created in 1986.

15 See, for example, Mason (1990).
16 Despite this demographic profile of Ontario, task force members saw fit to survey in detail only European and American midwifery systems, visiting England, Scotland, and Wales, as well as Denmark and the Netherlands. In the United States, members visited numerous midwifery practice sites including those staffed by nurse midwives and empirically trained midwives (TFIMO 1987, 39). No midwifery sites in either the Caribbean or the Philippines, the previous locations of midwifery practice for nearly half of those with training outside Canada, were visited during the investigations. While the TFIMO report claims to have reviewed material about midwifery in other countries, these are not named.
17 These arguments were being launched in response to an acrimonious debate in the midwifery community over the proposed nature of the Midwifery Education Program. Some midwives who remained opposed to regulation fought to retain the apprenticeship model and for the right to continue midwifery training outside of a formal midwifery education system. The authors of this quote spoke on behalf of the MTFO, a group historically aligned with the state-sponsored midwifery apparatus (Bourgeault 1996, 155). For a discussion of why Ontario midwives pursued legislation, see Van Wagner (2004).

Chapter 2: Midwifery in Ontario

1 Bourgeault (1996, 85) reports that while that funding for six liaison committee members was provided by the Council, nine midwives shared the disbursement.
2 Two white midwives who were working at the Povungnituk birth centre in Northern Quebec did make a submission to the curriculum development committee (CDC 1990, 51). The centre serves Inuit women in the North.
3 This policy may have stemmed from the overwhelming preference on the part of hospitals for midwives to be baccalaureate-prepared (Bourgeault 1996, 135).
4 This change in terminology represents an important discursive shift. I remember being corrected in 1995 by one midwifery activist when I used the term "foreign-trained" inasmuch as the "foreign" designation was seen to be a form of labelling people as "other." The apparent contradiction of a discursive shift to a less exclusionary terminology in the absence of inclusive practices that would give foreign-trained midwives access to practice was obvious to me at the time.
5 A search of the electronic newspaper article retrieval service Newscan yielded nearly daily articles on illegal immigration published between 1987 and 1993. References to the immigrants' Third World origins and to criminal activity are commonplace, and racist discourses about "tides," "floods," and "waves" of immigrants engulfing Canadian citizenry are frequent. See, for example, "Damming the Tide of Refugee Crime," *Toronto Sun,* 18 August 1993; "Tories Launch Blitz on Law and Order to Reassure Public," *Hamilton Spectator,* 4 November 1991; "Tough Talk on Immigrant Violence," 13 May 1991.
6 These trips included visits to a Native Friendship Centre in Timmins and community meetings in Moose Factory, Moosonee, and Attawapiskat on the James Bay coast between 29 March and 2 April 1992; a visit to the Akwesasne First Nation near Cornwall, Ontario, in June of 1992; a visit to Manitoulin Island in July 1992; and a visit to the Six Nations Reserve near Brantford, Ontario, in December 1992 (Ontario IRCM 1992d, 1992e, 1992f).
7 Stuart Hall also suggests the Freudian antecedents to the concept of "eating the Other," arguing that the process of identification requires that the "other" upon whom a given identity is contingent must be assimilated into the self. Hall (1996, 3) quotes Freud from *Mourning and Melancholia* on identification: "It behaves like a derivative of the first oral phase of organization of the libido in which the object that we long for is assimilated by eating and in that way annihilated as such."
8 See also Ward Churchill's analysis of attempts by New Age academics to appropriate First Nations religions and cultures. Churchill (1992, 210) aptly argues that while "the New Age can hardly be accused rationally of performing the conquest of the Americas, and its adherents go to great lengths in expressing their dismay at the methods used therein, they have clearly inherited what their ancestors gained by conquest, both in terms of resources and in terms of relative power."

9 Inderpal Grewal and Caren Kaplan criticize the use of terms such as "female genital mutilation," "excision," and "female circumcision" employed by feminist campaigns in the West to end the practice of surgically removing all or part of women's external genitalia. Such terminology, Grewal and Kaplan (1996, 10) argue, "is attached to a history of colonialism, linked to Enlightenment concepts of individuality and bodily integrity, medicalized notions of 'cleanliness' and 'health,' sexualized notions of the primacy of 'clitoral orgasm' and cultural organizations of pleasure." Referencing Isabelle Gunning's important work on the imperial effects of Western feminist interventions into these practices, Grewal and Kaplan (1994, 10) suggest the use of the term "genital surgeries" as one that avoids terminology that is either "ethnocentric and judgemental" or "misleadingly benign."

10 The admission that this issue was raised during the consultations is curiously excised from the most public document relating to the equity committee's meetings with "immigrant and refugee women," an article entitled "Midwifery Care for Immigrant and Refugee Women in Ontario" published in 1994 in *Canadian Woman Studies* (Ontario IRCM 1994).

11 The IRCM had opposed the appointment of any foreign-trained midwife who would not be eligible for registration upon passage of the Midwifery Act, a position that would have virtually guaranteed that immigrant midwives of colour would receive no representation on the Transitional Council (Eberts 27 July 1992).

12 The remaining 22 percent were from Eastern and Western Europe, Australia, and jurisdictions that were not identified.

13 In February 1995, I represented the Toronto Birth Centre at a meeting of the Community Advisory Committee of the PLA. Women of colour were outnumbered by white women, many of whom, unlike myself, were not representing community groups but rather were directly affiliated with the College of Midwives. The meeting was scrupulously scripted and choreographed and a dazzling display of white dominance in action; the atmosphere guaranteed that only the most aggressive unscheduled speakers managed to question the policy decisions being presented.

14 Minutes of the Community Advisory Committee to the Prior Learning Assessment of the Transitional Council of the College of Midwives of Ontario, 21 September 1993.

15 Project proposal from Association of Philippine Midwives, Summer 1994.

16 Minutes of the registration committee of the College of Midwives, 23 September 1994.

17 Minutes of the Community Advisory Committee to the PLA, 1 November 1994.

18 The CMO's Prior Learning Assessment project was renamed Prior Learning and Experience Assessment (PLEA) in December 1996.

19 The figures in this paragraph and in the one below are based on my interview on 11 March 1998 with CMO Registrar Robin Kilpatrick and PLEA Coordinator Jill Moriarty.

20 The unwillingness of the College of Midwives to release statistics about participation in the Prior Learning Assessment process with the numbers broken down by participants' country of origin makes any estimates of the racial composition of those who failed the English exam impossible to report.

21 Four out of eight PLA candidates interviewed, three of them native English speakers, mentioned the fast speaking pace of the person speaking on the audio-taped portion of the English exam. An exam based purely on a written response to taped speech, would, I believe, preclude the use of communicative strategies that are normally used in everyday life, such as asking people to repeat what they are saying, body language, and so on. Any testing that precludes the assessment of such communicative strategies may lack validity (Viete 1998).

22 One informant told me that the tape she heard included the phrase "broad as the side of a barn," an expression she determined to be largely North American in context.

23 The Toronto East Cultural Mentorship Initiative was a collaborative project undertaken by the Chinese Canadian Nurses Association of Ontario, the City of Toronto Department of Public Health, Toronto East General Hospital, and Riverdale Community Midwives. Designed to pursue "linguistically/culturally appropriate care ... for women who seek out midwives as their preferred caregivers during childbirth," as well as "to provide resource assistance for the ESL candidates" who apply to the PLA program in Toronto's eastern

areas, the Initiative provided bursaries to two candidates in the PLA program (Shroff 1997, 252). While financial aid was given to candidates, other forms of support were not forthcoming. Neither of the candidates funded by the project are currently working as midwives.

Chapter 3: Midwifery Tourism

1   It must be stressed that this number is merely an average. Some midwives attended thirty or forty births per year in this period, others attended relatively few. Also, owing to family responsibilities, travel, or study, midwives would often withdraw from practice for an extended period, during which other practitioners would take on larger caseloads (personal communication Christine Sternberg, RM, May 2000).
2   I am grateful to Margot Francis for suggesting this term.
3   The film, *Birth in the Squatting Position*, was produced in 1979 by two Brazilian physicians, Moyses and Claudio Paciornik, in their hospital in Curitiba, Brazil. In the Summer 1982 issue of the journal *Birth: Issues in Perinatal Care and Education*, the Paciorniks published an article that elaborated on the film, entitled "Rooming-in: Lessons Learned from the Forest Indians of Brazil." The article describes how the patients in their hospital follow the example of "our teachers, the Indian women out of the woods" (16).
4   Melissa Wright (2004, 370) has argued that political and corporate elites are now trying to transform the image of Ciudad Juárez, portraying assembly line maquiladora work done by young women as an "obsolete industrial tradition" in hopes of attracting a high-tech clientele to the region. Wright has demonstrated how both female industrial workers and the sex workers for whom the city is known have been made to "disappear" through kidnapping and legal harassment. The city has also been plagued by the murders and disappearances of hundreds of women and girls since 1993, giving rise to an active and outspoken coalition of women's movements demanding that local government and corporate elites solve not only these crimes but intervene in the numerous issues relating to violence against women in the region.
5   The Maternidad La Luz clinic in El Paso, Texas, for example, promises that students will attend approximately twenty-five to thirty-five births in a three-month "quarter" (Maternidad n.d.), nearly enough to fulfill the requirement (depending on the student's role at the birth) for attendance at the forty births required to sit the North American Registry of Midwives qualifying examination.

Chapter 4: "Ambassadors of the Profession"

1   Much of this vast literature in the United States and Canada arose simultaneously with the revival of lay midwifery in the late 1960s. For a review of the historical literature on midwifery see Litoff (1990). Recent work has achieved a more nuanced analysis of race, gender, class, and geography. See, for example, Wilkie (2003), Fraser (1998), and Borst (1995).
2   See, for example, Barbara Ehrenreich and Deirdre English's influential 1973 pamphlet *Witches, Midwives and Nurses*. See, as well, chapter 6 of Adrienne Rich's (1986) classic *Of Woman Born: Motherhood as Experience and Social Institution*.
3   For discussions of the disciplining and ultimate elimination of the black Southern midwife, see Susie (1988), Smith and Holmes (1996), and Fraser (1998).
4   As Judith Rooks (1997) demonstrates, wherever the practice of midwifery began to decline in the United States, maternal and infant mortality could be seen to increase.
5   The demise of Aboriginal midwifery has a complex history. In the first half of the twentieth century, a fair degree of medical pluralism existed wherein some First Nations women utilized the services of both traditional midwives and Canadian doctors. A rise in the incidence of complicated births, likely linked to conditions of colonization, precipitated demands in the 1940s by First Nations political leaders to challenge the Department of Indian Affairs' discriminatory policies relating to the access of First Nations Women to hospital maternity wards (Kelm 1998, 171).
6   In her history of midwifery in Canada, published as an appendix to the *Report of the Task Force on the Implementation of Midwifery*, Jutta Mason quotes from a privately published

monograph, M. Miyazaki's *My Sixty Years in Canada*, for which no date is given. From the context it can be understood that Mayazaki was a physician who practised in Vancouver in the 1930s. In a footnote, Mason (1987, 228) quotes Mayazaki as saying that "most Japanese people depended on Japanese midwives ... from Japan but who had no license to practice in B.C. ... Mrs. Watanabe was operating a rooming house so that Japanese women from the West Coast and country used to come to Vancouver a week before the expected date and stayed at her rooming house where Mrs. Watanabe delivered the baby and took care of the mother and baby ... 'I was called,' noted Watanabe, 'whenever these women had difficult cases.'"

7 For a discussion of Japanese-American midwives during internment in the United States during the Second World War, see Smith (1999).

8 There were some minor, but not uninteresting, exceptions to the trend toward hospitalization and physician-managed births. Childbirth with midwives continued, for example, well into the 1960s in outport Newfoundland communities (Benoit 1991). Although she offers only scant empirical evidence of this practice, Mason (1987) also suggests that midwife-attended births in Alberta Mennonite communities persisted well into the twentieth century.

9 For a review of these debates, see Mitchinson (1991).

10 This literature is vast. Some of the key works that inspired this movement and provided its proponents with empirical data upon which they could base their arguments include Kitzinger (1962), Arms (1975), Rothman (1982), Cohen and Estner (1983), and Oakley (1984).

11 In the past, nurse-midwives did train and practise in Canada but they worked mostly in rural areas and in the North. The University of Alberta School of Nursing began training nurse-midwives for rural areas and public health work in 1944, and in 1967 Dalhousie University initiated a program that included an internship in the Canadian North. Memorial University in Newfoundland also began a program in 1978 (Mason 1987). Prior to legislation in each province, Ontario, Alberta, and British Columbia instituted experimental nurse-midwife programs in tertiary-care hospitals (Harvey, Kaufman, and Rice 1995). Despite these initiatives, nurse-midwifery has not been embraced in Canada, where direct-entry midwifery has been adopted in all the provinces in which legislation has been effected.

12 See also Mason (1990).

13 "The Farm's" record of maternal and infant safety has been studied by public health scholars who examined the outcomes of 1,707 pregnancies of women delivered at the commune between 1971 and 1989. The conclusion was that for low-risk women home birth with lay midwives was not necessarily less safe than hospital birth with physicians (Durand 1992).

14 Gaskin is a far more pragmatic, scientific figure than her popular image conveys, developing in recent years highly efficacious obstetrical techniques lauded by both physicians and nurse-midwives (Rooks 1997).

15 Shorter's book was reissued in 1991 by Basic Books as *Women's Bodies*.

16 In her 1989 monograph "The dangers of professionalization," prepared as a discussion paper for the 22 November 1989 meeting of the Association of Ontario Midwives, midwifery critic Jutta Mason conjectures that "Louise Norman" was actually the pen name of midwife Theo Dawson.

17 Eastern Ontario has not remained without midwives. The College of Midwives of Ontario's list of midwifery practices dated 13 January 2004 lists seven midwifery practices in Eastern Ontario, including one serving Lanark County.

18 Within nursing, another female profession which has struggled to differentiate respectable from degenerate women, the trope of "proper dress" has a long history. See, for example, McPherson (1996). For an analysis of how dress has functioned as a racial signifier in nursing, see Marks (1994).

19 The practice of midwifery by lesbians is largely undocumented. I succeeded in finding only two references to or by lesbian midwives: an interview with well-known US lesbian midwife Anne Frye (Chester 1997) and an article by Inga Aarom (1996) entitled "Queer midwives," in *Hip Mama*, a parenting "zine" published in Oakland, California.

20 In February 1997, I delivered a paper at York University in which I outlined my preliminary analysis of racism in the midwifery movement. Two students of colour who were known to me signed comments on a sheet that was circulated among the one hundred or so participants, expressing their fervent opposition to my work and questioning why I would seek to undermine the newly established profession's credibility with my allegations.

Chapter 5: Narratives of Exclusion and Resistance of Women of Colour

1 It should be kept in mind that at the time of the interview, a given subject may have been in Canada for ten years, but she may have served on a board four or five years earlier and would have been, at the time of her service, a relative newcomer to Canada.

2 No such conflict of interest appeared to be perceived for the midwives who constituted the curriculum development committee or the registration committee, which formulated many of the policies governing the entry of midwives into practice subsequent to legislation, policies to which everyone would be subject.

3 People who served on some bodies related to midwifery implementation were granted government per diem payments intended to compensate them for lost work hours. However, they still needed to be in a position to negotiate absences from the workplace. Other committees, however, offered no such compensation and required members to attend daytime meetings.

4 In contrast to the immigrant women of colour interviewed for this study, a prominent Aboriginal woman had nothing but praise for her experience on a midwifery board. For this woman, exemption from midwifery legislation constituted a rare victory for Aboriginal women, and Aboriginal issues in relation to midwifery did receive significant attention in the years prior to legalization. In addition, midwifery activists cultivated a dialogue with Aboriginal women that was never in evidence in relation to immigrant women of colour.

5 This woman was a nurse in the racially diverse hospital mentioned below, and it is likely that many of the English-trained co-workers to whom she refers were women of colour.

6 While normally two midwives are required to be in attendance at a birth, registered midwives may engage suitably trained assistants as second attendants under certain circumstances.

7 I in no way wish to imply that I believe bureaucratic incompetence to be wholly benign. If people of colour experience delays, unresponsiveness, and mishandling of documents as racial prejudice, then a bureaucracy that expects to deal regularly with people of colour needs to be aware of how incompetence affects differently positioned groups. I would argue that an antiracist solution to this problem would be to apportion adequate resources and training to segments of a bureaucracy that are likely to deal with the public, so as not to foster racist exclusion through bureaucratic bungling.

8 Four out of the five women who spoke English as a second language held nursing jobs in which English fluency was indispensable. For only one woman, a very recent immigrant, did the interview pose a mild linguistic challenge.

9 An episiotomy is a surgical incision into the perineum intended to enlarge the birth canal during the second stage of labour. Its routine use has been in dispute for more than twenty years, and only recently has medical opinion begun to advocate a judicious rather than a liberal use of the procedure. See, for example, Lede, Belizan, and Carroli (1996).

10 For a distinctly Canadian example of this form of cross-cultural health care literature see Waxler-Morrison, Anderson, and Richardson (2005).

11 I can only offer a crude conjecture about the source of such a hesitation. The British National Health Service (NHS) has faced numerous charges of racism in recent years. The 8 percent of nurses and midwives in the NHS who are racialized minority people rise much more slowly in the nursing hierarchy than do their white colleagues (Beecham 1995) and few rise to managerial positions (Rashid 1990). A recent article that reported the testimonies about racism in the NHS offered by members of unions and professional associations claimed that "parents are telling their children not to follow them into the NHS. It has a bad reputation because of the way it treated people. Black health service workers are demoralised and disillusioned with the NHS and they are not convinced that their voices are being heard" (Watson 1998, 5). It would be difficult, I believe, for someone who has left

a racist employment situation to have to face its replica in the new country of residence, particularly when that country is touted, as is Canada, as a tolerant, multicultural state.

12 For a description of such initiatives, see Calliste (1996).

Conclusion: The Construction of Unequal Subjects

1 The Winter 2000 issue of the now-defunct *Association of Ontario Midwives Journal* carried an article by Vicki Van Wagner, now a faculty member at Ryerson University's Midwifery Education Program, reviewing a talk that I delivered at York University in 1997. Van Wagner (2000, 11) concedes that "thinking through Nestel's critique has been a valuable, if humbling push to look at how sometimes alternative movements make alternative oppressions." In a recent scholarly volume devoted to examining the re-emergence of Canadian midwifery (Bourgeault, Benoit, and Davis-Floyd 2004), four out of the fourteen chapters (not including my own) reference my work on racism in the Ontario midwifery movement.

2 In 2002, the College of Midwives of Ontario replaced their PLEA program with an International Midwifery Pre-registration Program (IMPP). This bridging program, run in cooperation with the Ryerson University Chang School of Continuing Education enjoys funding from the provincial government. The program provides language training and other courses that may streamline access to practice for internationally trained midwives.

3 For an historical overview of these initiatives, see Cullingworth (2003).

4 For important recent contributions to this field of research see Hunt (1999) and Roberts (1997).

5 In ten years of teaching childbirth education courses in urban hospitals in Toronto, I witnessed significant evidence of medical racism in which the reproductive lives of racialized minority women were the subject of pejorative commentary and women of colour frequently were the victims of aggressive and sometimes violent intervention. For descriptions of visible minority women's experiences of such racism, see Jawani (2001), Tudor (2001), Patel and Al-Jazairi (1997), and Jiminez (1991).

References

Aarom, Inga. 1996. Queer midwives. *Hip Mama* 9 (2nd quarter): 23.

Abate, G. 1998. Visible minorities will be majority by 2000. *Globe and Mail*, 18 June, A6.

Adams, T.L., and I.L. Bourgeault. 2003. Feminism and women's health professions in Ontario. *Women and Health* 38 (4): 73-90.

Agnew, V. 1996. *Resisting Discrimination: Women from Asia, Africa and the Caribbean and the Women's Movement in Canada*. Toronto: University of Toronto Press.

Ahmad, W.I.U. 1996. The trouble with culture. In *Researching Cultural Differences in Health*, ed. D. Kelleher and S. Hillier, 190-219. New York and London: Routledge.

Akbar, S., and D.J. Devoretz. 1993. Canada's demand for Third World highly trained immigrants 1976-1986. *World Development* 21 (1): 177-87.

Alarcon, N. 1996. Anzaldua's *Frontera:* Inscribing gynetics. In *Displacement, Diaspora, and Geographies of Identity*, ed. S. Lavie and T. Swedenburg. Durham, NC: Duke University Press.

Alexander, M.J. 1998. Imperial desire/sexual utopias: White gay capital and transnational tourism. In *Talking Visions: Multicultural Feminism in a Transnational Age*, ed. E. Shohat, 281-305. Cambridge, MA: The MIT Press.

Allemang, E., P. Armstrong, H. Armstrong, and F. Seddon. 1993. *Registration Project Report.* Transitional Council of the College of Midwives of Ontario.

Anthias, F., and N. Yuval-Davis. 1992. *Racialized Boundaries: Race, Nation, Gender, Colour and Class and the Anti-racist Struggle.* New York: Routledge.

Antunes, P., P.J.L. MacBride-King, and J. Swettenham. 2004. *Making a Visible Difference: The Contribution of Visible Minorities to Canadian Economic Growth.* Ottawa: Conference Board of Canada. Publication 570-04.

Anzaldua, G. 1987. *Borderlands/La Frontera: The New Mestiza.* San Francisco: Spinsters/Aunt Lute.

Arat-Koc, S. 1989. In the privacy of our own home: Foreign domestic workers as solution to the crisis in the domestic sphere in Canada. *Studies in Political Economy* 28: 33-58.

Arms, S. 1975. *Immaculate Deception: A New Look at Women and Childbirth in America.* San Francisco: San Francisco Book Company.

Arney, W.R. 1982. *Power and the Profession of Obstetrics.* Chicago: University of Chicago Press.

Arnup, K. 1994. *Education for Motherhood: Advice for Mothers in Twentieth-Century Canada.* Toronto: University of Toronto Press.

Association of Ontario Midwives. 1987a. *AOM Newsletter* 3 (3).

–. 1987b. *AOM Newsletter* 3 (4).

–. 1988. *AOM Newsletter* 4 (1).

–. 1990. *AOM Newsletter* 6 (1).

–. 1991. *AOM Newsletter* 7 (1).

–. 1993. *AOM 1991/1992 Report*.

–. n.d. *AOM Newsletter* 1 (1).

Azuh, M. 1998. *Foreign-Trained Professionals: Facilitating Their Contribution to the Canadian Economy*. Windsor: Windsor Women Working with Immigrant Women.

Badets, J., and L. Howatson-Leo. 1999. Recent immigrants in the workforce. *Canadian Social Trends* 52 (Spring): 16-22.

Bailey, A. 1998. Locating traitorous identities: Toward a view of privilege-cognizant white character. *Hypatia* 13 (3): 27-42.

Bailey, J.A.D. 2002. The Experiences and education of midwives in three Canadian provinces: Saskatchewan, Ontario and Nova Scotia. MA thesis, joint Women's Studies program, Mount Saint Vincent University, Dalhousie University, and St. Mary's University, Halifax, NS.

Bakan, A., and D. Stasiulis. 1994. Foreign domestic worker policy in Canada and the social boundaries of modern citizenship. *Science and Society* 58 (1): 7-33.

–. 1995. Making the match: Domestic placement agencies and the racialization of women's household work. *Signs* 20 (2): 303-35.

–. 1997. *Not One of the Family: Foreign Domestic Workers in Canada*. Toronto: University of Toronto Press.

Ball, R.E. 2004. Divergent development, racialised rights: Globalised labour markets and the trade of nurses: The case of the Philippines. *Women's Studies International Forum* 27 (2): 119-33.

Barbee, E. 1993. Racism and US nursing. *Medical Anthropology Quarterly* 7 (4): 346-62.

Barrington, E. 1985. *Midwifery Is Catching*. Toronto: New Canada Publishers.

Bauman, Andrea, Jennifer Blythe, Camille Kolotylo, and Jane Underwood. 2004. Immigration and emigration trends: A Canadian perspective. In *Building the Future: An Integrated Strategy for Nursing Human Resources*, ed. M. Downey. Ottawa: The Nursing Sector Study Corporation. www.buildingthefuture.ca/e/whatsnew/progressreport.

Baumgart, A.J., and M.M. Wheeler. 1992. The nursing work force in Canada. In *Canadian Nursing Faces the Future*, ed. A.J. Baumgart and J. Larsen, 45-70. St. Louis, MO: Mosby.

Beagan, B. 1998. Personal, public, and professional identities: Conflicts and congruences in medical school. PhD diss., University of British Columbia.

Beecham, L. 1995. Black and Asian nurses in the NHS report Harassment. *British Medical Journal* 311: 1247.

Benoit, C. 1991. *Midwives in Passage: The Modernization of Maternity Care*. St. John's: Institute of Social and Economic Research, Memorial University of Newfoundland.

Bhabha, H. 1994. *The Location of Culture*. New York: Routledge.

Biggs, L. 1990. "The case of the missing midwives": A history of midwifery in Ontario from 1795-1900. In *Delivering Motherhood: Maternal Ideologies and Practices in the 19th and 20th Centuries*, ed. K. Arnup, A. Levesque, and R.R. Pierson, 20-36. London: Routledge.

Bishop, R., and L. Robinson. 1998. *Night Market: Sexual Cultures and the Thai Economic Miracle*. New York: Routledge.

Borst, C. 1995. *Catching Babies: The Professionalization of Childbirth, 1870-1920*. Cambridge, MA: Harvard University Press.

Bourgeault, I. 1996. Delivering midwifery: An examination of the process and outcome of the incorporation of midwifery in Ontario. PhD diss., University of Toronto.

Boutilier, B. 1994. Helpers or heroines? The National Council of Women, nursing and "woman's work" in late Victorian Canada. In *Caring and Curing: Historical Perspectives on Women and Healing in Canada*, ed. D. Dodd and D. Gorham, 17-47. Ottawa: University of Ottawa Press.

Boyd, M. 1992. Gender, visible minority, and immigrant earnings inequality: Reassessing an employment equity premise. In *Deconstructing a Nation: Immigration, Multiculturalism and Racism in 90s Canada*, ed. V. Satzewich, 279-321. Halifax: Fernwood.

Boyer, H. 1992. Holy Family birth services. *Midwifery Today* 21 (2): 25-7.

Brodkin, K. 1998. *How Jews Became White Folks and What That Says about Race in America*. New Brunswick, NJ: Rutgers University Press.

Brown, T.C. 1997. The fourth member of NAFTA: The US-Mexico border. *Annals of the American Academy of Political and Social Science* 550: 105-21.

Brown, W. 1995. *States of Injury: Power and Freedom in Late Modernity.* Princeton: Princeton University Press.

Bruser, M. 1970. Midwife or matrician? *Canadian Medical Association Journal* 102 (11 April): 762.

Buckley, S. 1979. Ladies or midwives: Efforts to reduce infant and maternal mortality. In *A Not Unreasonable Claim: Women and Reform in Canada, 1880s to 1920s,* ed. L. Kealey, 148-63. Toronto: The Women's Press.

Burtch, B. 1994. *Trials of Labour: The Re-emergence of Midwifery.* Montreal and Kingston: McGill-Queen's University Press.

Burton, A. 1994. *Burdens of History: British Feminists, Indian Women and Imperial Culture, 1865-1915.* Chapel Hill, NC: University of North Carolina Press.

Butler, J. 2000. Appearances aside. *California Law Review* 88 (1): 55-63.

Butter, I., E. Carpenter, B.J. Kay, and R.S. Simmons. 1987. Gender hierarchies in the health labor force. *International Journal of Health Services* 17 (1): 133-49.

Caissey, I. 1994. Presentation to the City of North York's Community, Race and Ethnic Relations Committee, 13 October 1994. Toronto: Ontario Nurses Association.

Calliste, A. 1991. Canada's immigration policy and domestics from the Caribbean: The second domestic scheme. *Socialist Studies* 5: 136-68.

–. 1993. "Women of exceptional merit": Immigration of Caribbean nurses to Canada. *Canadian Journal of Women and the Law* 6 (1): 85-102.

–. 1996. Antiracism organizing and resistance in nursing: African-Canadian women. *Canadian Review of Sociology and Anthropology* 33 (3): 361-90.

–. 2000. Nurses and porters: Racism, sexism and resistance in segmented labour markets." In *Anti-Racist Feminism: Critical Race and Gender Studies,* ed. A. Calliste and G.J.S. Dei, 143-64. Halifax: Fernwood.

Canadian Nurses Association 1999. Registered nurses 1998 statistical highlights. www.cna-nurses.ca/pages/resources/stats/salary.

–. 2003. Fact Sheet: Nursing in Canada, June 2003. www.cna-aiic.ca.

Carpenter, M. 1993. The subordination of nurses in health care: Towards a social divisions approach. In *Gender Work and Medicine,* ed. E. Riska and K. Wegar, 95-130. London: Sage.

Carr, R. 1994. Crossing First World/Third World divides: Testimonial, transnational feminisms and the postmodern condition. In *Scattered Hegemonies: Postmodernity and Transnational Feminist Practices,* ed. I. Grewal and C. Kaplan, 153-72. Minneapolis: University of Minnesota Press.

Casa de Nacimiento. n.d. Pamphlet for prospective students. Postmarked 1997. El Paso, TX. Author's collection.

Chang, G. 1997. The global trade in Filipina workers. In *Dragon Ladies: Asian American Feminists Breathe Fire,* ed. S. Shah, 132-52. Boston: South End Press.

Chaudhuri, N., and M. Stroebel. 1992. *Western Women and Imperialism: Complicity and Resistance.* Bloomington: University of Indiana Press.

Chester, P. 1997. *Sisters on a Journey: Portraits of American Midwives.* New Brunswick, NJ: Rutgers University Press.

Chow, R. 1993. *Writing Diaspora.* Bloomington: Indiana University Press.

Choy, C.C. 2003. *Empire of Care: Nursing and Migration in Filipino American History.* Durham, NC: Duke University Press.

Choy, W. 1999. *Paper Shadows: A Chinatown Childhood.* Toronto: Viking.

Churchill, W. 1992. *Fantasies of the Master Race: Literature, Cinema and the Colonization of American Indians.* Monroe, ME: Common Courage Press.

Cohen, N.W., and L.J. Estner. 1983. *Silent Knife: Cesarean Prevention and Vaginal Birth after Cesarean.* Westport, CT: Bergin and Garvey.

College of Midwives of Ontario. 1994a. *Language and Prior Learning Assessment for Midwifery Project Phase III, Multifaceted Intensive Assessment.* Application for Access to Professions and Trades Demonstration Project Fund Part B: Project information. May 1994. Toronto.

–. 1994b. *Philosophy of Midwifery Care in Ontario.* Toronto.

–. 1994c. Policies on Prior Learning Assessment. Photocopy distributed at Prior Learning Assessment orientation session one. October 1994. Ontario Institute for Studies in Education, Toronto.

Cooke-Reynolds, M., and N. Zukewich. 2004. The feminization of work. *Canadian Social Trends* 72 (Spring): 22-9.

Cornish, M., E. McIntyre, A. Pask. 2001. Strategies for challenging discriminatory barriers to foreign credential recognition. *Canadian Labour and Employment Law Journal* 8: 17-53.

Couchie, C., and H. Nabigon. 1997. A path toward reclaiming Nishnawbe birth culture: Can the midwifery exemption clause for Aboriginal midwives make a difference? In *The New Midwifery: Reflections on Renaissance and Regulation,* ed. F. Shroff, 41-50. Toronto: Women's Press.

Cullingworth, J. 2003. Chronology of access to professions and trades initiatives and efforts in Ontario. Policy Roundtable Mobilizing Professions and Trades (PROMPT). Toronto.

Curriculum Design Committee on the Development of Midwifery Education in Ontario. 1990. *Report of the Curriculum Design Committee on the Development of Midwifery Education in Ontario.* Toronto.

Curtis, B., and C. Pajaczkowska. 1994. Getting there: Travel, time and narrative. In *Traveller's Tales: Narratives of Home and Displacement,* ed. G. Robertson, M. Mash, L. Tickner, and J. Bird. 199-215. New York: Routledge.

Daenzer, P. 1993. *Regulating Class Privilege: Immigrant Servants in Canada 1940s-1990s.* Toronto: Canadian Scholars Press.

Davidson, H.A. 1997. Territoriality among health care workers: Opinions of nurses and doctors towards midwives. EdD diss., University of Toronto.

Davis-Floyd, R.E. 1992. *Birth as an American Rite of Passage.* Berkeley: University of California Press.

Davis-Floyd, R.E., and C.F. Sargent, eds. 1997. *Childbirth and Authoritative Knowledge: Cross Cultural Perspectives.* Berkeley: University of California Press.

Daviss, B.A. 1999. From social movement to professional project: Are we throwing the baby out with the bathwater? MA thesis, Carleton University.

Davy, K. 1995. Outing whiteness: A Feminist/lesbian project. *Theatre Journal* 47 (2): 189-206.

Deere, C.D., P. Antrobus, L. Bolles, E. Melendez, P. Phillips, M. Rivera, and H. Safa. 1990. *In the Shadows of the Sun: Caribbean Development Alternatives and US Policy.* Boulder: Westview Press.

de Lauretis, T. 1984. *Alice Doesn't: Feminism, Semiotics, Cinema.* Bloomington: Indiana University Press.

Deloria, P.J. 1998. *Playing Indian.* New Haven: Yale University Press.

Denzin, N. 1994. The art and politics of interpretation. In *Handbook of Qualitative Research,* ed. N. Denzin and Y.S. Lincoln, 500-15. Thousand Oaks, CA: Sage.

Dickens, C. [1884] 1944. *Martin Chuzzlewit.* New York: Dodd.

Dominguez, V.R. 1995. Invoking racism in the public sphere: Two takes on national self-criticism. *Identities* 1 (4): 325-46.

Dua, E., L. FitzGerald, M. Gardner, D. Taylor, and L. Wyndels. 1994. *On Women Healthsharing.* Toronto: Women's Press.

Durand, A.M. 1992. The safety of home birth: The Farm study. *American Journal of Public Health* 82 (3): 450-3.

Dyer, R. *White.* 1997. New York: Routledge.

Eberts, M. 1992. Letter to A.R. Burrows, Director, Professional Relations Branch, Ontario Ministry of Health, from Chair of the IRCM. 27 July. Private collection.

Ehrenreich, B., and D. English. 1973. *Witches, Midwives and Nurses: A History of Women Healers.* New York: The Feminist Press.

Ehrenreich, B., and A.R. Hochschild. 2002. *Global Woman: Nannies, Maids and Sex Workers in the New Economy.* New York: Metropolitan Books, Henry Holt.

Enkin, M., M.J.N.C. Keirse, and I. Chalmers. 1995. *A Guide to Effective Care in Pregnancy and Childbirth.* New York: Oxford University Press.

Enloe, C. 1989. *Bananas, Beaches and Bases: Making Feminist Sense of International Politics.* London: Pandora.

Equay-wuk Women's Groups and Nishnawbe-Aski Nation. 1991. *Traditional Midwifery Practices and Recommendations.* Brief submitted to the Ontario Ministry of Health, September 1991.

Essed, P. 1991. *Understanding Everyday Racism: An Interdisciplinary Theory.* Newbury Park, NJ: Sage.

Etter-Lewis, G. 1993. *My Soul Is My Own: Oral Narratives of African American Women in the Professions.* New York: Routledge.

Fanon, F. 1963. *The Wretched of the Earth.* New York: Grove Press.

–. 1992. The Fact of Blackness. In *"Race," Culture and Difference,* ed. J. Donald and A. Rattansi, 220-40. London: Sage.

Fellows, M.L., and S. Razack. 1998. The race to innocence: Confronting hierarchical relations among women. *Journal of Gender, Race and Justice* 1 (Spring): 335-52.

Findlay, S. 1993. Problematizing privilege: Another look at the representation of "women" in feminist practice. In *And Still We Rise: Feminist Political Mobilizing in Contemporary Canada,* ed. L. Carty. 207-24. Toronto: Women's Press.

Fine, M. 1994. Working the hyphens: Reinventing self and other in qualitative research. In *Handbook of Qualitative Research,* ed. N. Denzin and Y.S. Lincoln, 70-82. Thousand Oaks, CA: Sage.

Fine, M., and L. Weis. 1996. Writing the "wrongs" of fieldwork: Confronting our own research/writing dilemmas in urban ethnographies. *Qualitative Inquiry* 2 (3): 251-74.

Flax, J. 1993. *Disputed Subjects: Essays on Psychoanalysis, Politics and Philosophy.* New York: Routledge.

–. 1998. *The American Dream in Black and White: The Clarence Thomas Hearings.* Ithaca, NY: Cornell University Press.

Ford, A.R. 1991. Equity committee report on a trip to Northwestern Ontario. *Ontario Gazette* 2 (2): 4-5.

–. 1992. The importance of an equity approach in consumer perspectives on midwifery. In *Shaping Midwifery: Report of the National Invitational Workshop on Midwifery Research and Evaluation,* McMaster University, 13-15 November 1992.

Ford, A.R., and V. Van Wagner. 2004. Access to midwifery: Reflections on the Ontario equity committee experience. In *Reconceiving Midwifery,* ed. I.L. Bourgeault, C. Benoit, and R. Davis-Floyd, 244-62. Montreal and Kingston: McGill-Queen's University Press.

Foucault, M. 1979. *Discipline and Punish: The Birth of the Prison.* New York: Vintage.

Frankenberg, R. 1993. *White Women, Race Matters: The Social Construction of Whiteness.* Minneapolis: University of Minnesota Press.

Fraser, G.J. 1998. *African American Midwifery in the South: Dialogues of Birth, Race and Memory.* Cambridge: Harvard University Press.

French, J. 1994. Hitting where it hurts most: Jamaican women's livelihoods. In *Mortgaging Women's Lives: Feminist Critiques of Structural Adjustment,* ed. P. Sparr, 165-82. London, UK: Zed Books.

Fynes, M.T. 1994. The legitimation of midwifery in Ontario 1960-1987. MA thesis, University of Toronto.

Gabriel, C. 1996. One of the Other? "Race," Gender, and the Limits of Official Multiculturalism." In *Women and Canadian Public Policy,* ed. J. Brodie, 173-95. Toronto: Harcourt Brace.

Galabuzi, G.-E. 2001. *Canada's Creeping Economic Apartheid: The Economic Segregation and Social Marginalization of Racialized Groups.* Toronto: CSJ Foundation.

Gaskin, I.M. 1978. *Spiritual Midwifery.* Summertown, TN: The Book Publishing Company.

Glazer, N. 1988. Overlooked, overworked: Women's unpaid and paid work in the health services "cost crisis." *International Journal of Health Services* 18 (1): 119-37.

Glenn, E.N. 1992. From servitude to service work: Historical continuities in the racial division of paid reproductive labor. *Signs* 18 (1): 1-43.

Goldberg, D.T. 1993. *Racist Culture: Philosophy and the Politics of Meaning.* Oxford, UK: Blackwell.

Goldman, B. 1988. Home birth: We did it, all of us. *Canadian Medical Association Journal* 139: 773.

Gonzales, A. 1992. Higher education, brain drain and overseas employment in the Philippines: Towards a differentiated set of solutions. *Higher Education* 23 (1): 21-31.

Gordon, S. 1991. *Prisoners of Men's Dreams: Striking Out for a New Feminine Future*. Boston: Little, Brown.

Gore, J.M. 1993. *The Struggle for Pedagogies: Critical and Feminist Discourses as Regimes of Truth*. New York: Routledge.

Gorham, D., and F.K. Andrews. 1990. *La Leche League: At the Crossroads of Medicine, Feminism, and Religion*. Chapel Hill: University of North Carolina Press.

Grewal, I. 1996. *Home and Harem: Nation, Gender, Empire and the Cultures of Travel*. Durham, NC: Duke University Press.

–. 1999. "Women's rights as human rights": Feminist practices, global feminism and human rights regimes in transnationality. *Citizenship Studies* 3 (3): 337-55.

Grewal, I., and C. Kaplan. 1994. *Scattered Hegemonies: Postmodernity and Transnational Feminist Practices*. Minneapolis: University of Minnesota Press.

–. 1996. "Warrior Marks": Global womanism's neo-colonial discourse in a multicultural context. *Camera Obscura* 39: 4-33.

Guendelman, S., and M. Jasis. 1992. Giving birth across the border: The San Diego-Tijuana connection. *Social Science and Medicine* 34 (4): 419-26.

Gunning, I. 1992. Arrogant perception, world-traveling and multicultural feminism: The case of female genital surgeries. *Columbia Human Rights Law Review* 23 (2): 189-248.

Hall, S. 1996. Introduction: Who needs "Identity"? In *Questions of Cultural Identity*, ed. S. Hall and P. du Gay, 1-17. Thousand Oaks, CA: Sage.

Haque, E. 1999. Reading immigration: Language, boundaries, space and nation. Unpublished course paper, Department of Sociology and Equity Studies, Ontario Institute for Studies in Education of the University of Toronto.

Harvey, S., K. Kaufman, and A. Rice. 1995. Hospital-based midwifery projects in Canada. In *Issues in Midwifery*, ed. T. Murphy-Black, 189-206. Edinburgh: Churchill Livingstone.

Henry, F., and E. Ginzberg. 1985. *Who Gets the Work? A Test of Racial Discrimination in Employment*. Urban Alliance on Race Relations and the Social Planning Council of Metropolitan Toronto.

Herman, E. 1996. All in the family: Lesbian motherhood meets popular psychology in a dysfunctional era. In *Inventing Lesbian Cultures in America*, ed. E. Lewin, 83-104. Boston: Beacon Press.

Hernandez, C. 1988. The Coalition of Visible Minority Women. In *Social Movements/Social Change*, ed. F. Cunningham, 157-68. Toronto: Between the Lines.

Heron, B. 1999. Desire for development: The education of white women as development workers. PhD diss., Department of Sociology and Equity Studies in Education, Ontario Institute for Studies in Education of the University of Toronto.

Higginbotham, E.B. 1992. African-American women's history and the metalanguage of race. *Signs* 17 (2): 251-79.

hooks, b. 1992. *Black Looks: Race and Representation*. Boston: South End Press.

Hunt, N.R. 1999. *A Colonial Lexicon of Birth Ritual, Medicalization and Mobility in the Congo*. Durham, NC: Duke University Press.

Hurst, L. 1999. Tragedy of immigrant brain reign. *Toronto Star*, 13 February, A1, A8.

Hurtado, A., and A.J. Stewart. 1997. Through the looking glass: Implications of studying whiteness for feminist methods. In *Off White: Readings on Race, Power and Society*, ed. M. Fine, L. Weis, L.C. Powell, and L. Mun Wong, 297-311. New York: Routledge.

International School of Midwifery. 1997. Jamaica Clinical Trip Information Sheet. Miami Beach, FL.

Isherwood, K. 1995. Independent midwifery in the United Kingdom. In *Issues in Midwifery*, ed. T. Murphy-Black. London: Churchill Livingstone.

Jacobs, J. 1996. *Edge of Empire: Postcolonialism and the City*. London: Routledge.

Jawani, Y. 2001. *Intersecting Inequalities: Immigrant Women of Colour, Violence and Health Care*. Vancouver: FREDA Centre for Research on Violence against Women and Children, Simon Fraser University.

Jiminez, M. 1991. Teniendo a mi hija (Having my baby). *Healthsharing* 12, 3 (Fall): 19-20.

Jordan, B. 1983. *Birth in Four Cultures: A Crosscultural Investigation of Childbirth in Yucatan, Holland, Sweden, and the United States*. Montreal and London: Eden Press.

Joyce, R.E., and C.L. Hunt. 1982. Philippine nurses and the brain drain. *Social Science and Medicine* 16: 1223-33.

Kaczorowski, J., C. Levitt, L. Hanvey, D. Avard, and G. Chance. 1998. A national survey of use of obstetric procedures and technologies in Canadian hospitals: Routine or based on existing evidence? *Birth* 25 (1): 11-18.

Kaplan, C. 1998. "Beyond the pale?": Rearticulating US Jewish whiteness. In *Talking Visions: Multicultural feminism in a transnational age*, ed. E. Shohat, 451-84. Cambridge: The MIT Press.

Kaye/Kantrowitz, M. 1996. Jews in the US: The rising costs of whiteness." In *Names We Call Home: Autobiography on Racial Identity*, ed. B. Thompson and S. Tyagi. New York: Routledge.

Kearney, M. 1991. Borders and boundaries of state and self at the end of empire. *Journal of Historical Sociology* 4 (1): 52-74.

Kelm, M.E. 1998. *Colonizing Bodies: Aboriginal Health and Healing in British Columbia 1900-1950*. Vancouver: University of British Columbia Press.

Kincaid, J. 1991. *Lucy*. New York: Plume.

Kitzinger, S. 1962. *The Experience of Childbirth*. London: Gollancz.

–. 1992. *Ourselves as Mothers*. London: Doubleday.

Klassen, P.E. 2001. *Blessed Events: Religion and Home Birth in America*. Princeton: Princeton University Press.

Kleiber, N., and L. Light. 1978. *Caring for Ourselves: An Alternative Structure for Health Care*. Vancouver: School of Nursing, University of British Columbia.

Kofman, E. 2004. Gendered global migrations: Diversity and stratification. *International Feminist Journal of Politics* 6 (4): 643-65.

Lather, P. 1992. Critical frames in educational research: Feminist and poststructural perspectives. *Theory into Practice* 31 (2): 87-99.

Lede, R.L., J.M. Belizan, and G. Carroli. 1996. Is routine use of episiotomy justified? *American Journal of Obstetrics and Gynecology* 174 (5): 1399-402.

Légère, E. 1995. Canadian multiculturalism and Aboriginal people: Negotiating a place in the nation. *Identities* 1 (4): 301-23.

Lian, J.Z., and R.D. Matthews. 1998. Does the vertical mosaic still exist? Ethnicity and income in Canada 1991. *Canadian Review of Sociology and Anthropology* 35 (4): 461-80.

Lipsitz, G. 1998. *The Possessive Investment in Whiteness: How White People Profit from Identity Politics*. Philadelphia: Temple University Press.

Litoff, J.B. 1978. *American Midwives, 1860 to the Present*. Westport, CT: Greenwood Press.

–. 1990. "Midwives and history." In *Women, Health and Medicine in America: A Historical Handbook*, ed. R.D. Apple, 443-58. New York: Garland.

Lum, J.M., and P.A. Williams. 2000. Professional fault lines: Nursing in Ontario after the regulated Health Professions Act. In *Care and Consequences: The Impact of Health Care Reform*, ed. D. Gustafson, 49-71. Halifax: Fernwood Publishing.

McCallum, W.T. 1979. The Maternity Center at El Paso. *Birth and the Family Journal* 6 (4): 259-66.

Macdonald, M.E. 1999. Expectations: The cultural construction of nature in midwifery discourse in Ontario. PhD diss., Department of Social Anthropology, York University.

McIntyre, A. 1997. *Making Meaning of Whiteness: Exploring Racial Identity with White Teachers*. Albany: SUNY Press.

McIsaac, E. 2003. Immigrants in Canadian cities: Census 2001 – What do the data tell us? *Policy Options* May 2003: 58-63.

MacKinnon, M. 1999. Give us your highly educated. *Globe and Mail*, 24 May, B1.

Macklin, A. 1992. Foreign domestic worker: Surrogate housewife or mail order servant? *McGill Law Journal* 37 (3): 681-760.

McNay, L. 1994. *Foucault: A Critical Introduction*. Cambridge, UK: Polity Press.

McPherson, K. 1996. *Bedside Matters: The Transformation of Canadian Nursing, 1900-1990*. Toronto: University of Toronto Press.

McRobbie, A. 1991. *Feminism and Youth Culture: From "Jackie" to "Just Seventeen."* Boston: Unwin Hyman.

Mani, L. 1998. *Contentious Traditions: The Debate on Sati in Colonial India.* Berkeley: University of California Press.

Marks, S. 1994. *Divided Sisterhood: Race, Class and Gender in the South African Nursing Profession.* New York: St. Martin's Press.

Martin, D. 1992. The midwife's tale: Old wisdom and a new challenge to the control of reproduction. *Columbia Journal of Gender and the Law* 3 (1): 417-48.

Martin, E. 1992. *The Woman in the Body: A Cultural Analysis of Reproduction.* Boston: Beacon Press.

Mason, J. 1987. A history of midwifery in Canada. In *Report of the Task Force on the Implementation of Midwifery in Ontario.* Toronto: Government of Ontario.

–. 1989. The dangers of professionalization: Part two. Talk delivered at Midwifery Task Force of Ontario meeting, "The dangers of professionalization," Toronto, February.

–. 1990. The trouble with licensing midwives. Ottawa: Canadian Research Institute for the Advancement of Women.

Maternidad La Luz Direct-Entry Midwifery Program. n.d. Mimeograph, postmarked 1997. El Paso, TX. Author's collection.

Matthews, R., and W. Thatcher. 1992. Ottawa responds. *Issue* [newsletter of the Midwifery Task Force of Ontario] 5 (4) and 6 (1): 21.

Mead, M. 1967. *Male and Female: A Study of the Sexes in a Changing World.* New York: William Morrow.

Melvin, Sara. 10 May 1991. Letter to Ontario Minister of Health Frances Lankin, on behalf of Equay-wuk (Women's Group). Private collection.

Midwifery Integration Planning Project. 1990. Minutes of meeting three. 5 December 1990.

Miller, L.M. 1997. The rhetorical construction of public policy: Public argument and the Florida legislature's debate over lay midwifery and homebirth 1950-1992. PhD diss., Indiana University of Pennsylvania.

Milligan, L.A. n.d. Letter from administrative/clinical director of Casa de Nacimiento, El Paso, TX, to prospective interns. Postmarked 1997. Author's collection.

Mitchinson, W. 1991. *The Nature of Their Bodies: Women and their Doctors in Victorian Canada.* Toronto: University of Toronto Press.

Mohanty, C. 1991. Cartographies of struggle: Third World women and the politics of feminism. In *Third World Women and the Politics of Feminism,* ed. C. Mohanty, A. Russo, and L. Torres, 1-47. Bloomington: University of Indiana Press.

Monk, H. 1994. Ontario midwifery in western historical perspective: From radicals to reactionaries in ten short years. Course paper for Athabasca University Women's Studies.

–. 1995. Institutional midwifery/organic midwifery – (Why) are they mutually exclusive? A systems analysis. Course paper for Athabasca University Women's Studies.

Morris, J. 1991. Letter to Ontario Minister of Health Frances Lankin. 7 May. Private collection.

Mosse, G.L. 1985. *Nationalism and Sexuality: Middle-Class Morality and Sexual Norms in Modern Europe.* Madison: University of Wisconsin Press.

Moure-Eraso, R. 1997. Back to the future: Sweatshop conditions on the Mexico/US border. *American Journal of Industrial Medicine* 31: 587-99.

MPL. 1993. Regulating Midwifery: Part of a New Beginning. 1993. *Pinoy sa Canada* 2, 3 (Winter): 2-3.

MTFO (Midwifery Task Force of Ontario). 1984. *Issue* [newsletter of the Midwifery Task Force of Ontario] 1, 2 (Winter): 84.

–. 1986. *Issue* [newsletter of the Midwifery Task Force of Ontario] (April): 11.

Murphy-Lawless, J. 1998. *Reading Birth and Death: A History of Obstetric Thinking.* Bloomington: University of Indiana Press.

Murray, M. 1999a. An immigrant's Catch-22 – No work, no experience. *Toronto Star,* 16 February, F1.

–. 1999b. MD can't even work as a nurse's aide. *Toronto Star,* 14 February, A1.

–. 1999c. Vet fights for level playing field. *Toronto Star*, 22 February, B1.

Nathan, Debbie. 1999. Death comes to the Maquilas: A border story. In *The Maquiladora Reader: Cross-Border Organizing since Nafta*, ed. R. Kamel and A. Hoffman, 27-30. Philadelphia: American Friends Service Committee.

National Council of Canadian Filipino Associations – Greater Toronto Region and Pinoy Sa Canada – Centre for Research, Education, Advocacy, Training and Employment. 1994. *Building Partnerships: Working toward Accreditation and Employment Equity, June 1993-June 1994*.

Natural Resources Canada. 2000. The Atlas of Canada: Nursing Resources. atlas.gc.ca/site/english/maps/health/resources/nursing/1.

Nestel, S. 1995. "Other mothers": Race and representation in natural childbirth discourse. *Resources for Feminist Research* 23 (4): 5-19.

–. 1996-7. "A new profession to the white population in Canada": Ontario midwifery and the politics of race. *Health and Canadian Society* 4 (2): 315-41.

Ng, R. 1988. *The Politics of Community Services: Immigrant Women, Class and State*. Toronto: Garamond.

Ng, R., and A. Estable. 1987. Immigrant women in the labour force: An overview of present knowledge and research gaps. *Resources for Feminist Research* 16 (1): 29-33.

Norman, L. 1983. Survival tactics for midwives. *Issue* [newsletter of the Ontario Association of Midwives] 3 (2): 7.

Oakley, A. 1984. *The Captured Womb: A History of the Medical Care of Pregnant Women*. Oxford: Basil Blackwell.

O'Neil, J., and P. Kaufert. 1990. The politics of obstetric care: The Inuit experience. In *Births and Power*, ed. W.P. Hendwerker, 53-86. Boulder, CO: Westview Press.

–. 1995. Irniktakpunga! Sex determination and the Inuit struggle for birthing rights in Northern Canada. In *Conceiving the New World Order*, ed. F. Ginsburg and R. Rapp, 59-73. Los Angeles: University of California Press.

Ong, A. 1995. Women out of China: Traveling tales and traveling theories in postcolonial feminism. In *Women Writing Culture*, ed. R. Behar and D. Gordon, 350-72. Berkeley: University of California Press.

–. 1996. Cultural citizenship as subject making: Immigrants negotiate racial and cultural boundaries in the United States. *Current Anthropology* 37 (5): 737-62.

Ong, P., and T. Azores. 1994. The migration and incorporation of Filipino nurses. In *The New Asian Immigration in Los Angeles and Global Restructuring*, ed. P. Ong, E. Bonacich, and L. Cheng, 164-95. Philadelphia: Temple University Press.

Ontario. Ministry of Training, Colleges and Universities. 2002. *The Facts Are In! A Study of the Characteristics and Experiences of Immigrants Seeking Employment in Regulated Professions in Ontario*. Toronto. Summer. www.edu.gov.on.ca/eng/document/reports/facts02.pdf.

Ontario Interim Regulatory Council on Midwifery (IRCM). 1990a. Ontario's Interim Regulatory Council on Midwifery. *Ontario Gazette* 1 (1).

–. 1990b. *Report on the Visit to Ottawa*. 25 April. Toronto: IRCM.

–. 1991a. Aboriginal women's group adopts resolution on midwifery profession. *Ontario Gazette* 2 (1): 3.

–. 1991b. Equity committee meets special groups face to face to research midwifery needs. *Ontario Gazette* 2 (1): 5.

–. 1991c. *Report of a Trip to Northwestern Ontario Made by the Equity Committee*. October. Toronto.

–. 1992a. Equity committee report examines midwifery and immigrant women. *Ontario Gazette* 3 (2): 2-3.

–. 1992b. Midwifery needs of disabled women and teen mothers under study. *Ontario Gazette* 3 (1): 2-3.

–. 1992c. *Minutes*. 24 November. Toronto.

–. 1992d. *Report of a Trip to Timmins and the James Bay Coast Made by the Equity Committee March 29-April 2, 1992*. Toronto.

–. 1992e. *Report of a Visit by the Equity Committee to the Six Nations Reserve, Ohsweken, Ontario, December 14, 1992*. Toronto.

–. 1992f. *Report of a Visit to the Prison for Women in Kingston and Akwesasne First Nation by the Equity Committee June 22-23, 1992.* Toronto.

–. 1992g. Equity Committee. *Presentation to the Royal Commission on Aboriginal Peoples.* 2 November 1992. Toronto.

–. 1993a. IRCM's equity committee was unique among the health professions. *Ontario Gazette* 3 (1): 10-1.

–. 1993b. *Midwifery and Immigrant and Refugee Women: Report of the Equity Committee.* Toronto.

–. 1994. Equity Committee. Midwifery care for immigrant and refugee women in Ontario. *Canadian Woman Studies* 14 (3): 83-6.

Ontario Native Women's Association. 1991. Position on Aboriginal midwifery. Position paper, 1 August. Toronto Birth Centre archives.

Ontario Nurse-Midwives Association. n.d. *For your information.* Pamphlet. Toronto.

Oppenheimer, J. 1990. Childbirth in Ontario: The transition from home to hospital in the early twentieth century. In *Delivering Motherhood: Maternal Ideologies and Practices in the 19th and 20th Centuries,* ed. K. Arnup, A. Levesque, and R.R. Pierson, 51-74. London: Routledge.

Ornstein, M. 1996. *Ethno-Racial Inequality in Metropolitan Toronto: Analysis of the 1991 Census.* Toronto: Access and Equity Centre of the Municipality of Metropolitan Toronto.

Ortega, H. 1991. Crossing the border for bargain medicine: Findings of the Primary Health Care Review in Ambos Nogales. *Carnegie Quarterly* 35: 1-4.

Ortin, E.L. 1990. The brain drain as viewed by an exporting country. *International Nursing Review* 37 (5): 340-44.

Paciornik, M., and C. Paciornik. 1983. Rooming-in: Lessons learned from the forest Indians of Brazil." *Birth: Issues in Perinatal Care and Education* 10, 2 (Summer): 115-19.

Papps, E., and M. Olssen. 1997. *Doctoring Childbirth and Regulating Midwifery in New Zealand: A Foucauldian Perspective.* Palmerston North, NZ: The Dunsmore Press.

Parreñas, Rhacel Salazar. 2001. *Servants of Globalization: Women, Migration and Domestic Work.* Stanford, CA: Stanford University Press.

Patel, S., and I. Al-Jazairi. 1997. Colonized wombs. In *The New Midwifery: Reflections on Renaissance and Regulation,* ed. F. Shroff, 51-81. Toronto: Women's Press.

Pateman, B. 1998. Computer-aided qualitative data analysis: The value of NUD*IST and other programs. *Nurse Researcher* 5 (3): 77-89.

Pierson, R.R., and N. Chaudhuri. 1993. The Mainstream Women's Movement and the Politics of Difference. In *Strong Voices.* Vol. 1 of *Canadian Women's Issues,* ed. R.R. Pierson, M.G. Cohen, P. Bourne, and P. Masters, 186-214. Toronto: James Lorimer.

–. 1999. *Nation, Empire, Colony: Historicizing Gender and Race.* Bloomington: Indiana University Press.

Policy Roundtable Mobilizing Professions and Trades. 2004. *In the Public Interest: Immigrant Access to Regulated Professions in Today's Ontario.* Toronto.

Pollock, G. 1994. Territories of desire: Reconsiderations of an African childhood. In *Traveller's Tales: Narratives of Home and Displacement,* ed. G. Robertson, M. Mash, L. Tickner, and J. Bird. 63-92. New York: Routledge.

Pope, C. 2001. Babies and borderlands: Factors that influence Sonoran women's decisions to seek prenatal care in southern Arizona. In *Geographies of Women's Health,* ed. I. Dyck, N. Davis Lewis, and S. McLafferty, 143-58. New York: Routledge.

Pratt, G. 1999. From registered nurse to registered nanny: Discursive geographies of Filipina domestic workers in Vancouver, BC. *Economic Geography* 75 (3): 215-36.

Pratt, M.L. 1992. *Imperial Eyes: Travel Writing and Transculturation.* New York: Routledge.

Prell, R. 1999. *Fighting to Become Americans: Jews, Gender, and the Anxiety of Assimilation.* Boston: Beacon Press.

Preston, V., and W. Giles. 1997. Ethnicity, gender and labour markets in Canada: A case study of immigrant women in Toronto. *Canadian Journal of Urban Research* 6 (2): 135-59.

Ransom, J.S. 1997. *Foucault's Discipline: The Politics of Subjectivity.* Durham, NC: Duke University Press.

Rashid, A. 1990. Asian doctors and nurses in the NHS. In *Health Care for Asians,* ed. B. McAvoy and L.J. Donaldson, 40-56. Oxford: Oxford University Press.

Rattansi, A. 1994. Western racisms, ethnicities, and identities in a "postmodern" frame. In *Racism, Modernity, and Identity on the Western Front,* ed. A. Rattansi and S. Westwood, 15-86. Cambridge, UK: Polity Press.

Razack, S. 1998a. *Looking White People in the Eye: Gender, Race, and Culture in Courtrooms and Classrooms.* Toronto: University of Toronto Press.

–. 1998b. Race, space and prostitution: The making of the bourgeois subject. *Canadian Journal of Women and the Law* 10: 338-76.

–. 1999. Making Canada white: Law and the policing of bodies in the 1990s. *Canadian Journal of Law and Society* 14 (1): 159-83.

–. 2000. "Your place or mine?": Transnational feminist collaboration. In *Anti-racist Feminism: Critical Race and Gender Studies,* ed. A. Calliste and G.J.S. Dei, 39-53. Halifax: Fernwood.

Rich, A. 1986. *Of Woman Born: Motherhood as Experience and Social Institution.* New York: W.W. Norton.

Roberts, D. 1997. *Killing the Black Body: Race, Reproduction, and the Meaning of Liberty.* New York: Pantheon.

Rodriguez, N. 1996. The battle for the border: Notes on autonomous migration, transnational communities and the state. *Social Justice* 23 (3): 21-23.

Romalis, S. 1985. Struggle between providers and recipients: The case of birth practices. In *Women, Health and Healing,* ed. V. Oleson and E. Lewin, 174-208. New York: Tavistock.

Roman, L. 1993. White is a color! White defensiveness, postmodernism and anti-racist pedagogy. In *Race, Identity, and Representation in Education,* ed. C. McCarthy and W. Crichlow, 71-88. New York: Routledge.

–. 1997. Denying (white) racial privilege: Redemption discourses and the uses of fantasy. In *Off White: Readings on Race, Power and Society,* ed. M. Fine, L. Weis, L.C. Powell, and L. Mun Wong, 270-82. New York: Routledge.

Rooks, J.P. 1997. *Midwifery and Childbirth in America.* Philadelphia: Temple University Press.

Rosaldo, R. 1989. Imperialist nostalgia. *Representations* 26: 107-22.

Ross-Kerr, J.C., and M. Wood. 2002. *Canadian Nursing.* 4th ed. Toronto: Mosby Canada.

Rothman, B.K. 1982. *In Labor: Women and Power in the Birthplace.* New York: W.W. Norton.

Rushing, B. 1993. Ideology in the re-emergence of North American midwifery. *Work and Occupations* 20 (1): 46-67.

Said, E. 1993. *Culture and Imperialism.* New York: Alfred A. Knopf.

Salzinger, L. 2003. *Genders in Production: Making Workers in Mexico's Global Factories.* Berkeley: University of California Press.

Sandoval, C. 1997. Theorizing white consciousness for a post-empire world: Barthes, Fanon, and the rhetoric of love. In *Displacing Whiteness: Essays in Social and Cultural Criticism,* ed. R. Frankenberg, 86-106. Durham, NC: Duke University Press.

Sargent, C.F., and G. Bascope. 1997. Ways of knowing about birth in three cultures. In *Childbirth and Authoritative Knowledge,* ed. E. Davis-Floyd and C.F. Sargent, 183-208. Berkeley: University of California Press.

Sassen, S. 1988. *The Mobility of Labor and Capital: A Study in International Investment and Labor Flow.* Cambridge: Cambridge University Press.

Schatz, D.M. 1992. *Report on the Admission Process Pre-registration Program Midwifery.* Toronto: Michener Institute for Applied Health Sciences.

Schick, C. 1998. By virtue of being white: Racialized identity formation and the implications for anti-racist pedagogy. PhD diss., Department of Sociology and Equity Studies, Ontario Institute for Studies in Education of the University of Toronto.

Schutte, O. 1998. Cultural alterity: Cross-cultural communication and feminist theory in North-South contexts. *Hypatia* 13 (2): 53-72.

Scully, D. 1994. *Men Who Control Women's Health: The Miseducation of Obstetrician-Gynecologists.* New York: Teachers College Press.

Seabrook, J. 1996. *Travels in the Skin Trade: Tourism and the Sex Industry.* London: Pluto Press.

Sears, D. 1997. Notes of a "Colored Girl ...": 32 short reasons why I write for the theatre. Program notes for the Canadian Stage Company/Nightwood Theatre production of *Harlem Duet,* written and directed by Djanet Sears, 27 October-29 November 1997, Canadian Stage Company, St. Lawrence Centre.

Sedgwick, E.K. 1990. *The Epistemology of the Closet*. Berkeley: University of California Press.

Sedivy-Glasgow, M. 1992. Nursing in Canada. *Canadian Social Trends* 24 (Spring).

Sharpe, M. 1993. Journeying with my inner map. Course paper submitted to the Department of Adult Education, Ontario Institute for Studies in Education of the University of Toronto.

Shearer, M. 1989. Maternity Patients' Movements in the United States, 1820-1985. In *Effective Care in Pregnancy and Childbirth*, ed. M. Enkin, J. Keirse, and I. Chalmers, 110-29. New York: Oxford University Press.

Shildrick, M. 1997. *Leaky Bodies and Boundaries: Feminism, Postmodernism and (Bio)ethics*. London: Routledge.

Shohat, E., and R. Stam. 1994. *Unthinking Eurocentrism: Multiculturalism and the Media*. London: Routledge.

Shorter, E. 1991. *Women's Bodies*. New York: Basic Books.

Shroff, F.M. 1997. All petals of the flower: Celebrating diversity of Ontario's birthing women within first-year midwifery curriculum. In *The New Midwifery: Reflections on Renaissance and Regulation*, ed. F. Shroff, 261-310. Toronto: Women's Press.

Sibley, D. 1995. *Geographies of Exclusion*. London: Routledge.

Silvera, M. 1989. *Silenced: Talks with Working Class Caribbean Women about Their Lives and Struggles as Domestic Workers in Canada*. Toronto: Sister Vision.

Silverman, K. 1986. Fragments of a fashionable discourse. In *Studies in Entertainment: Critical Approaches to Mass Culture*, ed. T. Modleski. Bloomington: Indiana University Press.

Sleeter, C. 1996. White silence, white solidarity. In *Race Traitor*, ed. N. Ignatiev and J. Garvey, 257-65. New York: Routledge.

Smith, M.C., and L.J. Holmes. 1996. *Listen to Me Good: The Life Story of an Alabama Midwife*. Columbus: Ohio State University Press.

Smith, S.L. 1999. Women health workers and the color line in the Japanese American "Relocation Centers" of World War II. *Bulletin of the History of Medicine* 73 (4): 585-601.

Soja, E. 1996. *Thirdspace: Journeys to Los Angeles and Other Real-and-Imagined Places*. Cambridge, MA: Blackwell.

Spivak, G.C. 1988. Can the Subaltern Speak? In *Marxism and the Interpretation of Culture*. ed. C. Nelson and L. Grossberg, 271-313. Urbana, IL, and Chicago: University of Chicago Press.

–. 1999. *A Critique of Postcolonial Reason: Toward a History of the Vanishing Present*. Cambridge, MA: Harvard University Press.

Starr, P. 1982. *The Social Transformation of American Medicine*. New York: Basic Books.

Stasiulis D., and A. Bakan. 2003. *Negotiating Citizenship: Migrant Women in Canada and the Global System*. Houndsmill, UK: Palgrave.

Statistics Canada. 1990. *Women in Canada: A Statistical Report*. 2nd ed. Cat. no. 89-503E. Ottawa: Ministry of Supply and Services.

–. 1991a. *Census Metropolitan Districts, Statistics Canada: 1991 Employment Equity Data Report on Designated Groups*. www.statcan.ca.

–. 1991b. *Provincial Employment Equity Ontario*, Part 2. www.statcan.ca.

–. 1995. *Women in Canada: A Statistical Report*. 3rd ed. Housing, Family and Social Statistics Division: Target groups project. Ottawa: Statistics Canada.

–. 1999. 1996 Census Nation Tables. www.statcan.ca.

–. 2002. *Ethnic Diversity Survey: Portrait of a Multicultural Society*. Cat. no. 89-593-XIE. Ottawa: Statistics Canada.

–. 2003. *2001 Census*. Ethnocultural Portrait of Canada: Profile Ontario. www.statcan.ca.

–. 2004. *2001 Census*. Ethnocultural Portrait of Canada: Subprovincial. www.statcan.ca.

Staub, M.E. 1999. "Negroes are not Jews": Race, Holocaust consciousness and the rise of Jewish neo-conservatism. *Radical History Review* 75: 3-27.

Stewart, D., and R. Pong. 1997. *Summary Report of the 1996 Survey of First-year Students of the Midwifery Education Program and a Comparison of the 1993, 1994, 1995 and 1996 Cohorts of First-year Students*. Working paper W97-9. September. Northern Health Human Resources Research Unit, Laurentian University and Lakehead University.

–. 1998. *A Profile of the 1997 Cohort of Applicants to the Midwifery Education Program and a Comparison of the 1993, 1994, 1995, 1996, and 1997 Cohorts of Applicants.* Working paper W98-5. March. Centre for Rural and Northern Health Research, Laurentian University and Lakehead University.

Stoler, A.L. 1995. *Race and the Education of Desire: Foucault's History of Sexuality and the Colonial Order of Things.* Durham, NC: Duke University Press.

Sullivan, D.A., and R. Weitz. 1988. *Labor Pains: Modern Midwives and Home Birth.* New Haven, CT: Yale University Press.

Susie, D.A. 1988. *In the Way of Our Grandmothers: A Cultural View of Twentieth Century Midwifery in Florida.* Athens, GA: University of Georgia Press.

Sutton, W., M. Cheetham, H. Krieger, and C. Sternberg. 1993. Free-standing birth centres: The Toronto Birth Centre model. *The Canadian Journal of Ob/Gyn and Women's Health Care* 5 (4): 473-77.

Takagi, D.Y. 1996. Maiden voyage: Excursion into sexuality and identity politics in Asian America. In *Queer Theory/Sociology,* ed. S. Seidman. Cambridge, MA: Blackwell.

Task Force on Access to Professions and Trades in Ontario. 1989. *Access!* Toronto: Ontario Ministry of Citizenship.

Task Force on the Implementation of Midwifery in Ontario. 1987. *Report of the Task Force on the Implementation of Midwifery in Ontario.* Toronto: Ontario Ministry.

Terry, C., and L. Calm Wind. 1994. Do-dis-seem. *Canadian Woman Studies* 14 (3): 77-82.

Thomas, B.L. 1993. *Report on Traditional Aboriginal Midwifery in Ontario, Phase One.* Ontario Native Women's Organization, 13 July 1993.

Thomson, R.G. 1997. Feminist theory, the body, and the disabled figure. In *The Disability Studies Reader,* ed. L.J. Davis, 279-92. New York: Routledge.

Tollefson, J.W. 1991. *Planning Language, Planning Inequality: Language Policy in the Community.* London: Longman.

Tran, K. 2004. Visible minorities in the labour force: 20 years of change. *Canadian Social Trends* (Summer): 7-11.

Treichler, P. 1990. Feminism, medicine, and the meaning of childbirth. In *Body/Politics,* ed. M. Jacobus, E.F. Keller, and S. Shuttleworth, 113-38. New York: Routledge.

Trinh, T.M. 1989. *Woman, Native, Other: Writing Postcoloniality and Feminism.* Bloomington: Indiana University Press.

–. 1991. *When the Moon Waxes Red: Representation, Gender and Cultural Politics.* New York: Routledge.

Tudor, T. 2001. The politics of reproduction: Childbirth, health and culture in Greater Vancouver, British Columbia. MA thesis, Department of Sociology and Anthropology, Simon Fraser University.

Tyson, H. 1991. Outcomes of 1001 midwife-attended home births in Toronto, 1983-1988. *Birth* 18 (1): 14-19.

–. 2001. Who gets to be a midwife? Who gets midwifery care? In *Midwifery in Canada: Directions for Research,* ed. J. Kornelson. Proceedings from the National Invitational Workshop on Midwifery Research, 9-11 May. Vancouver. Vancouver: British Columbia Centre for Excellence in Women's Health.

Umansky, L. 1996. *Motherhood Reconceived: Feminism and the Legacies of the Sixties.* New York: New York University Press.

United Nations. Economic and Social Affairs Population Division. 2003. *Trends in Total Migrant Stock: The 2003 Division.* www.un.org/esa/population/publications/migstock/2003TrendsMigstock.pdf.

van Dijk, T.A. 1993a. Analyzing racism through discourse analysis: Some methodological reflections. In *Race and Ethnicity in Research Methods,* ed. J.H. Stanfield II and R.M. Dennis, 92-134. Newbury Park, CA: Sage.

–. 1993b. *Elite Discourse and Racism.* Newbury Park, CA: Sage.

Van Wagner, V. 1988a. How to speak about midwifery issues. *The Midwifery Issue* [newsletter of the Midwifery Task Force of Ontario] 2, 2 (Winter): 11-14.

–. 1988b. Women organizing for midwifery in Ontario. *Resources for Feminist Research* 17 (3): 136-39.

–. 2000. Book review: *A New Profession to the White Population in Canada: Ontario Midwifery and the Politics of Race,* by Sheryl Nestel. *Association of Ontario Midwives Journal* 6 (4): 10-11.

–. 2004. Why legislation? Using regulation to strengthen midwifery. In *Reconceiving Midwifery,* ed. I.L. Bourgeault, C. Benoit, and R. Davis-Floyd, 71-90. Montreal and Kingston: McGill-Queen's University Press.

Viete, R. 1998. Culturally sensitive and equitable access of oral English for overseas-qualified teacher trainees. *Journal of Intercultural Studies* 19 (2): 171-86. In Expanded Academic [database online] Article no. A53459976 [accessed 28 October 1999].

Waite, G. 1993. Childbirth, lay institution building, and health policy: The Traditional Childbearing Group, Inc. of Boston in a historical context. In *Wings of Gauze: Women of Color and the Experience of Health and Illness,* ed. B. Blair and S.E. Cayleff, 202-25. Detroit: Wayne State University Press.

Ware, V. 1992. *Beyond the Pale: White Women, Racism and History.* London: Verso.

Warwick, A., and D. Cavallaro. 1998. *Fashioning the Frame: Boundaries, Dress and the Body.* Oxford, UK: Berg.

Watson, S. 1998. Tackling racism could end recruitment crisis. *Nursing Standard* 13, 13-15 (December-January): 5.

Waxler-Morrison, N., J. Anderson, and E. Richardson. 2005. *Cross-Cultural Caring: A Handbook for Health Professionals.* Vancouver: UBC Press.

Weigman, R. 1995. *American Anatomies: Theorizing Race and Gender.* Durham, NC: Duke University Press.

Weitz, R. 1987. English midwives and the Association of Radical Midwives. *Women and Health* 12 (1): 79-89.

Wells, L. 1998. Consulting to black-white relations in predominantly white organizations. *Journal of Applied Behavioral Science* 34 (4): 392-96.

Wertz, R., and D. Wertz. 1989. *Lying-in: A History of Childbirth in America.* New Haven, CT: Yale University Press.

Wetherell, M., and J. Potter. 1992. *Mapping the Language of Racism: Discourse and the Legitimation of Exploitation.* New York: Columbia University Press.

White, H. 1981. The value of narrativity in the representation of reality. In *On Narrative,* ed. W.J.T. Mitchell, 1-23. Chicago: University of Chicago Press.

Wilkie, L. 2003. *The Archaeology of Mothering: An African American Midwife's Tale.* New York: Routledge.

Winkup, J.L. 1998. Reluctant redefinition: Medical dominance and the representation of midwifery in CMAJ 1966-1997. MA thesis, Department of Anthropology, University of Guelph.

Wright, M. 2001. Feminine villains, masculine heroes and the reproduction of Ciudad Juárez. *Social Text 69* 19 (4): 19-113.

–. 2004. From protests to politics: Sex work, women's worth and Ciudad Juárez modernity. *Annals of the Association of American Geographers* 94 (2): 369-86.

Wu, Y.S. 1998. Domestic workers in the underground economy: The lack of civil rights protections. *Poverty and Race* [online newsletter of the Poverty & Race Research Action Council]. March-April. www.prrac.org.

Index

Aboriginal communities, 3, 27, 31, 45
  discursive strategies concerning, 148-51
  midwives, 27, 39, 45-51, 88-9, 172n11,
    178ch4n5
  representatives on midwifery bodies,
    128-36, 180n4
  as source of traditional knowledge, 3,
    49-50, 176n8
access to registration. *See* registration
access to training
  effects of cost, 64-5, 138
  equity issues, 27, 28, 30, 32, 52
  exclusionary policies, 39-41, 52-3, 54,
    56-68
  TFIMO recommendations, 32-6, 40
Allemang, Elizabeth, 56
AOM. *See* Association of Ontario Midwives
  (AOM)
Armstrong, Hugh, 56
Armstrong, Pat, 56
Association of Ontario Midwives (AOM),
  27, 28, 31, 38, 70-1, 95
  outreach committee, 27-30
Association of Philippine Midwives, 58-9

Barrington, Eleanor, 93
British National Health Service, 180n11
British-trained midwives, 22, 91, 144-5,
  175n8

Canadian Medical Association, 90
Canadian Nurses Association, 174n3
CDC. *See* Curriculum Design Committee
  on the Development of Midwifery
  Education in Ontario (CDC)
Ciudad Juárez (Mexico), 74-5, 77,
  178ch3n4
clientele
  marginalized groups, 27, 31-2

white, 139-40
  women of colour, 26, 31, 41
clothing. *See* modes of dress
College of Midwives, 53, 181n2
  bureaucratic inefficiencies, 65-6, 67
  See also language issues; Prior Learning
    and Experience Assessment project
    (PLEA); registration
College of Nurses Ontario survey, 32-3
Committee for More Midwives, 96
constructions of respectability, 7, 9, 84-8,
  95-116
consumers. *See* clientele
costs of training, 64-5, 138
counterculture midwives, 84-6, 96-104
cross-border childbirth, US-Mexico, 71,
  74-82, 172n11, 178ch3n5
Curriculum Design Committee on the
  Development of Midwifery Education in Ontario (CDC), 39-40

Daviss, Betty-Anne. *See* Putt, Betty-Anne
direct-entry midwifery, 6, 171n4. *See also*
  midwifery tourism
discrimination. *See* exclusionary practices
doctors, 5, 88, 89-90, 172n8
domestic workers, 18-19, 21, 22
dress codes. *See* modes of dress

Eberts, Mary, 31, 38
educational requirements, 39-40, 171n2
  clinical experience, 41, 60-1, 70-1, 82-3
  language exams, 59-60, 62-4, 138, 156,
    177n20-n22
  Michener Institute Pre-registration
    Program, 40, 46, 64, 66, 96, 97, 98,
    141
  Midwifery Education Program (MEP),
    104-24, 146-7, 172n11

See also access to training; Prior Learning and Experience Assessment project (PLEA)
El Paso (Texas), 74, 75, 76, 77, 178ch3n5
Equay-wuk Women's Group, 45, 46
exclusionary practices, 4-5, 7-8, 37-8, 67-8, 85
  anti-immigrant discourse, 18-19, 34-5, 163-4, 176n5
  assessment of foreign credentials, 35, 40, 56-68, 137-8
  claimed philosophical differences, 33-5, 84-6, 96-104, 137, 143-5
  constructions of respectability, 7, 9, 84-8, 95-116
  costs, 64-5, 138
  against counterculture midwives, 84-6, 96-104
  language issues, 59-60, 62-4, 138, 151-2, 156, 177n20-n22
  marginalization on midwifery bodies, 38-9, 128-36
  racist sentiment, 18-19, 34-5, 66-7, 99-100, 116-24, 140, 151-3, 176n5
  resistance to, 155-9
  role in establishment of midwifery, 4-5, 8, 17-18, 24-6, 42-5, 51-2, 84-5, 91-104, 160-6
  systemic racism, 65-7, 116-24
  training access policies, 39-40, 52-3, 54, 56-68

family responsibilities, 100-1, 108
feminist projects, 5, 29, 31-2, 52, 67, 70, 95, 146, 160
  imperialism and, 7-8, 71-2, 73, 165-6
Filipino midwives, 58-9
Fine, Michelle, 126
First Nation communities. *See* Aboriginal communities
foreign-trained midwives, 32-4, 38, 41-2, 174n4-n5
  assessment of credentials, 35, 40, 56-68, 137-8
  Association of Ontario Midwives and, 27-8, 29
  British-trained, 22, 91, 144-5
  exclusion from training opportunities, 39-41, 52-3, 54, 56-68
  term definition, 174n4, 176n4
  TFIMO report, 32-6, 38, 40
  See also exclusionary practices; immigrant midwives; nurse-midwives
Frye, Anne, 110-11

Gaskin, Ina May, 170n14
  Spiritual Midwifery, 92-3
genital surgeries, 51, 177n9
Guatemala, midwifery tourism, 76

Health Professions Legislation Review (HPLR), 27, 175n13
Hernandez, Carmencita, 58
home birth, 22, 33-5, 70, 179n13
  experience of midwives of colour, 33-4, 137, 143
Home Birth Task Force, 22, 23
hospitals, ethnic diversity, 138-9
HPLR. *See* Health Professions Legislation Review (HPLR)
Humber College/Women's College Hospital Childbirth Educators Multidisciplinary Certificate Program, 105

immigrant midwives, 23-4, 174n5
  Interim Regulatory Council on Midwifery (IRCM) and, 51-3
  lack of access to information, 41, 140, 142, 146-50
  white immigrant experiences, 154, 164
  See also foreign-trained midwives; immigrant women; midwives of colour
immigrant women, 32, 51
  domestic workers, 18-19, 21, 22
  nurses, 174n5-n6, 175n8
  role in social mobility of First World women, 18-19, 21, 163
  See also immigrant midwives; midwives of colour
immigrants, 33, 54-6, 66-7, 174n5-n6
  anti-immigrant discourse, 18-19, 34-5, 163-4, 176n5
  barriers to professional practice, 54-6, 163
  See also immigrant midwives
IMPP (International Midwifery Pre-registration Program), 181n2
integration programs, 35-6, 40-5
Interim Regulatory Council on Midwifery (IRCM), 38-9, 42-50, 177n11
  equity committee, 44-53
  interviewees, 42-3, 50-2
International Midwifery Pre-registration Program (IMPP), 181n2
interviewees
  immigrants who pursued registration, 140-50
  Interim Regulatory Council on Midwifery members, 42-3, 50-2

Midwifery Education Program students, 105-23
nurse-midwives who did not seek registration, 136-40
white midwives, 98-104, 175n12
women on midwifery boards/bodies, 128-36, 180n1
See also research methodology
IRCM. *See* Interim Regulatory Council on Midwifery (IRCM)

Jamaica
midwifery tourism, 76, 77
nurses from, 174n5-n6
Jews, 10-11

Lanark Midwifery Support Association, 98
language issues, 59-60, 62-4, 79-80, 138, 151-2, 156, 177n20-n22
Laurentian University. *See* Midwifery Education Program (MEP)
lay midwifery. *See* direct-entry midwifery
legal liability, 139-40
legislation, 6, 28, 175n9
lesbian midwives, 107, 108-11, 116, 179n19

McMaster University. *See* Midwifery Education Program (MEP)
Maloney, Teresa, 30
marginalized people, 44-5
and research methodologies, 125-7, 161-2
See also Aboriginal communities; immigrant women; women of colour
MEP. *See* Midwifery Education Program (MEP)
Mexico-US border clinics, 71, 74-82, 172n11, 178ch3n4-n5
Michener Institute Pre-registration Program, 40, 46, 64, 66, 96, 97, 98, 141
midwifery, 5-6
history in Canada, 88-91, 168-9, 178ch4n5-179n11
history in the United States, 87-8
See also midwifery movement
Midwifery Act (1990), 6, 28, 175n9
Midwifery Education Program (MEP), 104-5, 146-7, 172n11
construction of respectability, 105-16
students of colour, 116-24
Midwifery Integration Planning Project (MIPP), 39, 41
midwifery movement, 91
chronology, 168-9

construction of respectability, 7, 9, 84-8, 95-104
discursive strategies, 51-3, 84, 85-6, 91-104, 143-4
role of women of colour, 4, 26-7, 38-9, 51-3, 57-9
socio-economic characteristics, 6, 23-4, 38-9, 43, 146-7, 151-3, 157, 159
suppression of counterculture influences, 84, 91-104
midwifery regulation, 172n9
Aboriginal issues, 39, 45-51
legislation, 6, 28, 175n9
prelegislation stages, 27-36, 95
See also registration
Midwifery Task Force of Ontario (MTFO), 27, 31, 34
midwifery tourism, 8, 28-9, 69-70, 72-3, 76-9, 82-3
language issues, 79-80
US-Mexico border clinics, 71, 74-82, 172n11, 178n5
midwives
Aboriginal communities, 27, 39, 45-51, 88-9, 178n5
British-trained, 22, 91, 144-5, 175n8
with counterculture philosophies, 84-6, 96-104
with disabilities, 113-14
from Jamaica, 174n5-n6
lesbians, 107, 108-11, 116, 179n19
from Philippines, 58-9, 174n5-n6
rural regions, 28, 29-30, 96-8, 179n17
United States, 87-8, 91
See also foreign-trained midwives; immigrant midwives; nurse-midwives; midwives of colour; student midwives
midwives of colour, 4, 57
access to Ontario experience/ information, 41, 140, 142, 146-50
employment, 24, 26, 41-2, 137-9
experience with home birth, 33-4, 137, 143
interactions with white midwives, 23, 24-5, 99-100
involvement in PLA/PLEA process, 57-9
resistance to exclusionary practices, 155-9
students, 116-24
See also exclusionary practices; foreign-trained midwives; immigrant midwives; nurse-midwives
midwives with disabilities, 113-14
migrant women. *See* immigrant women

MIPP. *See* Midwifery Integration Planning Project (MIPP)
modes of dress, 84, 100, 103-4, 106-8, 179n18
MTFO. *See* Midwifery Task Force of Ontario (MTFO)

National Council of Women, 89
Nestel, Sheryl, 10-14
    reception of her research, 13, 15, 172n15, 180n20, 181n1
    See also research methodology
Nishnawbe-Aski Nation, 46
Norman, Louise, 94-5, 179n16
nurse-midwives, 32-3, 40, 163, 174n3, 174n5, 175n8, 179n11
    midwives of colour, 21, 24, 25-6, 32-6, 136-45, 146-50, 174n5
    Ontario Nurse-Midwives Association, 22-3, 27
    reluctance to pursue registration, 26, 41-2, 136-40
    stereotypes/racist discourse concerning, 25, 34-5
    support for home birth, 33-4, 137, 143
nursing, 19-21, 89-90, 174n3, 175n8, 179n18. *See also* nurse-midwives

OAM. *See* Ontario Association of Midwives (OAM)
ONMA. *See* Ontario Nurse-Midwives Association (ONMA)
Ontario Association of Midwives (OAM), 23, 27. *See also* Association of Ontario Midwives (AOM)
Ontario Native Women's Association, 45-6
Ontario Nurse-Midwives Association (ONMA), 22-3, 27. *See also* Association of Ontario Midwives (AOM)

Philippines
    midwifery tourism, 76
    midwives from, 58-9, 174n5-n6
physical appearance. *See* modes of dress
physicians, 5, 88, 89-90, 172n8
PLA/PLEA process. *See* Prior Learning and Experience Assessment project (PLEA)
prelegislation midwifery, 22-35
Prior Learning and Experience Assessment project (PLEA), 57, 61, 64, 65-6, 164
    early stages (PLA), 56-60, 129
    experiences of interviewees, 141-50, 153, 156-8
    role in credentialing midwives of colour, 61-2, 65-6

Prior Learning Assessment project (PLA), 56-7
    community advisory committee, 57-60, 129
    See also Prior Learning and Experience Assessment project (PLEA)
Pustil, Judi, 91-2
Putt, Betty-Anne, 3, 28, 29, 171n1

racialized minority women. *See* Aboriginal communities; immigrant women; midwives of colour; women of colour
racism, 18-21, 66-7
    American midwifery and, 86-8
    definitions, 37-8
    See also exclusionary practices
Re-Birth (newspaper), 92
registration, 61
    assessment of foreign credentials, 35, 40, 56-68, 137-8
    clinical experience requirements, 41, 60-1, 70-1, 82-3
    educational requirements, 40, 171n2
    integration programs, 35-6, 40-5
    reluctance of nurse-midwives to pursue registration, 26, 41-2, 136-40
regulation. *See* midwifery regulation; registration
research methodology, 8-10, 172n16
    information letter for research participants, 167-8
    interview cohorts, 127-9, 136-7, 140-2
    interview schedules, 169-70
    interviews, 14-15, 117, 161, 173n16-n22
    marginalized groups/individuals and, 125-7, 161-2
    poster for research participants, 168
    See also interviewees; Nestel, Sheryl
respectability. *See* constructions of respectability
rural midwives, 28, 29-30
    Eastern Ontario, 96-8, 179n17
Russell, Jesse, 39, 44-5, 48
Ryerson Polytechnic University. *See* Midwifery Education Program (MEP)

Schwartz, Allan, 97
Seddon, Freda, 56
sexual identity, 107, 108-11
Shorter, Edward, 94
spiritual beliefs, 100, 102-3, 114-15
student midwives, 11-12, 104-6
    disabilities, 113-14
    experience of racism, 116-24

physical appearance, 106-8
sexual identity, 107, 108-11, 116, 120
socio-economic pressures, 111-13

TAAM. *See* Toronto Association of
Aspiring Midwives (TAAM)
Task Force on Access to Professions and
Trades in Ontario (TFAPTO), 55, 163
Task Force on the Implementation of
Midwifery in Ontario (TFIMO), 30-1
College of Nurses Ontario survey, 32-3
hearings and submissions, 31, 97
report, 32-4, 35-6, 38, 40, 70, 176n16
TFAPTO. *See* Task Force on Access to
Professions and Trades in Ontario
(TFAPTO)
TFIMO. *See* Task Force on the Implementa-
tion of Midwifery in Ontario (TFIMO)
Third World
midwifery clinics, 76, 77
as source of traditional knowledge,
28-9, 72-3
term definition, 172n10
women, 17-18
See also immigrants; midwifery tourism
Toronto Association of Aspiring Midwives
(TAAM), 146-7
Toronto Birth Centre, 172n16
Toronto East Cultural Mentorship
Initiative, 177n23

traditional knowledge
Aboriginal childbirth, 3, 49-50
Third World childbirth, 28-9, 72-3
training. *See* access to training; educational
requirements; student midwives
Transitional Council of the College of
Midwives, 53-4, 56, 128

United States
history of midwifery, 87-8, 91
US-Mexico border clinics, 71, 74-82,
172n11, 178ch3n5

Van Wagner, Vicki, 84, 85, 92, 181n1
visible minorities. *see* Aboriginal communities; midwives of colour; women
of colour

Weis, Lois, 126
women of colour
as clients, 26, 31
political organization and, 31-2
presence on midwifery councils, 38-9,
51-4, 128-36
term definition, 172n7
See also immigrant women; midwives
of colour
Wu-Lawrence, Betty, 58